T0198016

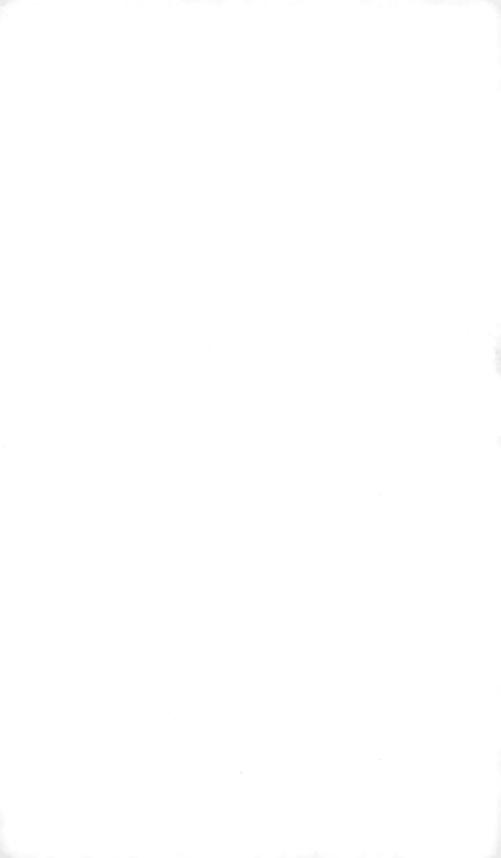

Women and Medicine

Third Edition

Beatrice Levin

The Scarecrow Press, Inc.
Lanham, Maryland, and London
2002

SCARECROW PRESS, INC.

Published in the United States of America
by Scarecrow Press, Inc.
4720 Boston Way, Lanham, Maryland 20706
www.scarecrowpress.com

4 Pleydell Gardens, Folkestone
Kent CT20 2DN, England

First edition © 1980 by Beatrice S. Levin. Metuchen, NJ: Scarecrow Press. ISBN 0-8108-1296-7
Second edition ©1988 by Beatrice Levin. Lincoln, NE: Media Publishing. ISBN 0-939644-28-2

British Library Cataloguing-in-Publication Information Available

Library of Congress Cataloging-in-Publication Data

Levin, Beatrice.
    Women and medicine / Beatrice Levin.— 3rd ed.
      p. cm.
    Includes bibliographical references and index.
    ISBN 0-8108-4238-6 (alk. paper)
    1. Women in medicine. 2. Women in medicine—Biography. 3. Women in medicine—United States. 4. Sexism in medicine—United States. I. Title.
    R692 .L49 2002
    610'.82'0973—dc21   2001055045

Contents

Preface   v

Acknowledgments   vii

1   The Dinosaur Is Twitching: 1
Famous Firsts

2   To Be a Doctor in America: 9
Overcoming Obstacles

3   Shattering the Glass Ceiling: 23
Surgeons General and Presidents' Doctors

4   Historical Perspectives: 35
Midwives and Doctors around the Globe

5   Women on the March: 77
Civil War Heroines

6   Pioneers, O Pioneers!:   89
Then and Now

7   One University's Contributions: 129
Those Remarkable Johns Hopkins Women

8   Oh, Brave New World: 143
Nobel Prize Winners in Medicine

9   Women's Proper Place: 167
Our Biological Selves

10   A Peaceful Revolution: 183
      The Fight for Birth Control

11   What Was the Doctor Wearing?:   189
      From White Coats to Space Suits

      Bibliography   197

      Index   201

      About the Author   205

Preface

The greatest changes in technology of the past century were not in information and computing but in medicine and health. The most significant changes have been in the role of women in medicine and science.

Increasing enrollments of women in medical schools and in practice have markedly influenced medical education and research. In 2000, 25 percent of practicing physicians were women. More than 50 percent of incoming medical students are female, and at some prestigious schools women constitute half the first-year class. Compare these statistics with 1970 when the average enrollment of women in medical school was 9 percent.

In 1900 life expectancy in the United States was only forty-seven years; by 2000 it was around seventy-seven years. A century ago, disinfectants, anesthesia, and vaccination had become commonplace, but doctors were only beginning to accept the germ theory of disease. Consider the dazzling developments of a century of pharmaceuticals: antibiotics, penicillin, and antituberculosis drugs. In the first seventy years of the century, doctors could prescribe drugs to conquer typhoid, tetanus, and diphtheria. Readily at hand were antiviral agents against many formerly deadly ills such as yellow fever, polio, measles, German measles, and other life-threatening diseases. We have witnessed a revolution in oncology, chemotherapies, microsurgery, plastic surgery, heart surgery, and appendectomies.

In 2000 Vivian Pinn, director of the Federal Office of Research on Women's Health (established in 1990), claimed, "We are modifying explanations of what the norms in medicine should be because they were developed by men, for and about men."

For decades, scientists limited studies of heart disease and cancer to men, theorizing that men were more likely to develop those diseases earlier and "males were easier to recruit into studies." But just as many women died of heart disease as men, though women die ten years later. Heart disease in the twenty-first century may be the leading killer of postmenopausal women. Breast cancer and gynecological cancer strike greater fear in the hearts of women than heart attacks. When women learned that seven out of every ten women were at risk to develop breast cancer, many willingly became volunteers in breast cancer studies.

By 1996 the National Institute of Health, responding to complaints by women's advocacy groups and congresswomen, provided a federal grant of roughly $662 million to enroll volunteers and doctors to study women's risk factors in breast and colon cancer, heart disease, and fractures. One phase of the study tested the effects of hormones, vitamins, minerals, and diet; the other observed women over a period of time to determine their rate of heart disease, breast and colon cancer, and osteoporosis (a condition causing brittle bones) in the general population. Should women take hormone replacement therapy (estrogen) and risk breast cancer? Or refuse such therapy and risk osteoporosis?

In the last three decades of the century, women geniuses have contributed to the development of major new drugs against ulcers, mental problems, cancer, and heart disease. Women are playing a role in every aspect of medicine, especially the care of the elderly and infirm.

Nobel Prize winner Dr. Rosalyn Yalow was convinced there had long been "marked professional discrimination against women and other disadvantaged groups for admission to medical schools . . . and strong social pressures to discourage them from professional careers."

The women's health movements and the increasing number of women in medical school have created a quiet revolution in medical education, reshaping curriculums and clinical experiences. Women physicians recognize that their practices require not more mechanization of medicine, but more humanization, and doctors who offer not only orders, but hope, courage, and compassion. Good health is the promise of grace, a zest for life, joy in the morning, exuberance in work and play, and a gift that calls for gratitude. In this human community, good medicine may be available to all, and good medical training available to all who qualify.

Acknowledgments

Words are inadequate to express my appreciation to my husband, Dr. Franklyn K. Levin, for his enduring patience, support, and love for more than half a century and for his meticulous proofreading of three editions of *Women and Medicine*.

Interviews at Hadassah Hospital in Israel with Chloe Tal, Florella Magora, Kadari Avishag, and Mayera Glassman took place in the early 1980s. *Hadassah Magazine* provided the photo of Chloe Tal. The New York Infirmary supplied photos of Elizabeth Blackwell and Marie Zakrzewska.

Also in the 1980s in Houston, Texas, I interviewed Helen Mintz Hittner, a specialist in pediatric ophthalmology, Hilde Bruch, a specialist in eating disorders, and Joycelyn Elders. The photos of Joycelyn Elders were taken at a Planned Parenthood meeting.

In Hawaii, I interviewed Dr. Ruth Kleinfeld Lenny and Professor Roy G. Smith. Dr. Smith taught Saudi women medical students at an extension of the University of Hawaii School of Public Health in Dammam, Saudi Arabia.

Dr. Estelle Ramey at Georgetown University School of Medicine, Washington, D.C., gave me copies of her articles with permission to quote from them and a photograph.

In 1972 Margery Scott-Young led me on a tour of the Rachel Forster Hospital in Sydney, Australia, and invited me to her home. She gave me news clippings and a booklet about Susannah Hennessy O'Reilly, who helped found the New Hospital for Women and Children in Sydney in 1921.

Jana Moser, a Czech plastic surgeon, studied in Texas in 1975 at the Galveston Shrine Institute for Burned Children where I interviewed her.

The *Florida Times-Union* sent me a photo of Anne Lavall Sundstrom with permission for using it in this book.

Though Marie Valdes-Dapena had eleven children while carrying on a full-time profession, she took the time to write me twice and gave me permission to quote her. The first of the annual family photos she sent me disappeared, and she generously and promptly sent me the one that appears in this book.

Barbara Jean Gretsch at forty-five, after rearing seven children, began a medical education against tremendous odds. Her husband sent me her photo in cap and gown with her delighted family. Gretsch's photo appeared in the *Saturday Evening Post* (March 1981, p. 126) and was sent to me at my request with permission to publish. When the second edition of *Women and Medicine* was published, the Gretsch family purchased a dozen autographed copies.

Stella Robertson has kept me updated on her significant research since we met some decades ago at a conference of the Society of Exploration Geophysicists. She also provided a photo.

I include a brief biography of my niece, Dr. Jacqueline Wolf, with photo provided by her mother, Carolyn Sachs.

Cicely Williams, a gentle lady, corresponded with me, describing her appreciation for the years she studied pellagra at Charity Hospital in New Orleans, Louisiana. (She asked if the climate in my home city of Houston was as humid as in New Orleans.) She added some memories she had failed to recall for her biographer, Ann Dally, who wrote *The Story of a Doctor* (1968, Gollancz, London). Williams sent me the autographed photo that appears in this book.

Dr. Rosalyn Yalow edited the biography I wrote of her and sent me photos for the second edition of *Women and Medicine.*

Meharry Medical School provided the photo of Dr. Dorothy Brown.

Jennifer Niebyl sent a biography, some published papers, and a photo.

Loyal friends, Doctors Annette and Paul Vigny of the Institute Curie, Paris, provided the pictures of Marie Curie.

Dr. Antonia Novello sent me her photo and a resume.

Some passages from *Office Hours: Day and Night*, by President Kennedy's doctor, Janet Travell (1968, New American Library, Inc., New York), are reprinted by arrangement with the publishers. I interviewed her in Galveston, Texas, and she provided me with her photo.

Greek-American magazines have published a number of my articles on Greek women in medicine. The chapter "Historical Perspectives" is based on my lectures.

For permission to quote from Ruth Fox Hume's *Florence Nightingale* (1964), I'm indebted to Random House, New York. Photo courtesy of Culver Pictures, Inc., London.

Permission to quote from the *Women's Medical Journal—Fifty Years Ago—A Retrospect* (October 1893) was granted for my use of references to Elizabeth Blackwell, Harriot Hunt, and Marie Zakrzewska, and from Case Western Reserve Medical Alumni Bulletin (1969, 33: 4), Harry D. Piercy, "Marie Zakrzewska, Class of 1856."

For a portrait of Elizabeth Garrett and James Anderson and some biographic insights, I'm indebted to Louisa Garrett's biography of her mother published by Faber & Faber.

For material on *The Life of Sophia Jex-Blake, M.D.*, by Margaret Todd, I owe a debt to Macmillan, London (1918).

I studied Dorothy C. Wilson's *Stranger and Traveler: The Story of Dorothea Dix* (1975, Little, Brown and Co., Boston, Toronto) and David Gollaher's *Voice for the Mad: The Life of Dorothea Dix* (1995, The Free Press, Simon and Schuster, Inc., New York). For the picture of Dorothea Dix, I am grateful to Macmillan Books, New York, 1910.

Nanette Kass Wenger provided her photograph and replied to my requests for an update of an earlier article I wrote.

Biographical information about Alexandria Adler came from the Alfred Adler Mental Hygiene Clinic in New York.

Helen Hittner graciously consented to being interviewed in Houston, Texas.

Dr. Siddiqa Pasha provided photos and information about her hospital.

Mary Edwards Walker was the subject of a *Literary Digest* article (4/15/1919): "Dr. Mary Walker's Eccentric Dress Drew Attention from Her Real Achievements."

My articles on Bickerdyke and Clara Barton were previously published in 1990 by the Cowles History Group (602 S. King St., Leesburg, VA 22075).

Jo Manton, author of *Elizabeth Garrett Anderson* (1965, Methuen, London) gave me permission to quote from her biography of a life that revealed great courage.

I used Mary Putnam Jacobi's writings edited by the Women's Medical Association of New York (1925, G.P. Putnam).

Material on Dr. Florence Rena Sabin is based on Albert Q. Maisel's *Dr. Sabin's Second Career* (1947, Survey Graphic, 36: 138–140) and Lawrence S. Kubie's "Florence Rena Sabin" in *Perspectives in Biology and Medicine* (5: 306–314) and on letters from her students. Photo of Sabin provided by Johns Hopkins University.

The Passano Foundation sent me the 1948 photo of Helen Taussig.

Photos and references to Gerty Radnitz Cori and Rita Levi-Montalcini came from Washington University Public Relations (St. Louis, Missouri) with permission to publish.

Between 1990 and 2001, Brenda Edwards, Nancy Dickey, Eleanor Wallace, Marcella Willock, Florence Haseltine, and Susan Band Horowitz each graciously and promptly responded to my request for a bio and a photo.

The California Medical Association in 1971 provided a bio and a photo of Roberta Fenlon.

Sometime around 1950, Brigitte Horney responded to my request for a photo of her mother, Karen Horney, and gave permission to publish it. For some of the biographical material, I am indebted to W. W. Norton Co., Inc., New York, publisher of many of Karen Horney's books.

The Sloan Foundation Science Series provided permission to quote from Levi-Montalcini's *In Praise of Imperfection: My Life and Work* (1988, Basic Books, New York). Washington University provided the photo.

Burroughs-Wellcome supplied the information on Gertrude Elion. Photo courtesy of Will and Deni McIntyre.

Permission came from Walker and Co. to quote from Beatrice Bishop Berle's *A Life in Two Worlds*, and Funk and Wagnall granted permission for use of Rosalie

Slaughter Morgan's Iranian holiday material, while Robert Hale of London sent permission for "fair use" of Morgan's *A Woman Surgeon.*

For the chapter on Marie Nyswander, I referred to newspapers and magazines from 1956 to 1969. Her 1956 book, *The Drug Addict as Patient* (Greun and Stratton), was wonderful, as was Nat Hentoff's *A Doctor among the Addicts* (1968, Rand McNally, New York).

The photo of Margaret Sanger was provided by Planned Parenthood. I referred to Sanger's *Autobiography* (1938, Norton, New York), and *Margaret Sanger: A Biography of the Champion of Birth Control* by Madeline Gray (1979, Richard Marek Publishers, New York).

The photo of Gertrude Stein and the Cone sisters was provided by the Baltimore Museum of Art.

Harcourt, Brace, and Jovanovich granted permission for the use of the photo of Marie Stopes and brief quotes from Ruth Hall's *Passionate Crusader: The Life of Marie Stopes* (1977) and Marie Stopes's *Married Love* (1918).

The Carnegie Institution, Washington, D.C., provided the photo of Nobel-Prize winner Barbara McClintock.

Like Frances Oldham Kelsey's work on thalidomide and other drugs, Nancy Wexler's crusade against Huntington's disease has been widely documented. Wexler's office supplied her photo and information with permission to publish.

Alain and Micheline Ferrandon drove me from Paris to Tubingen for the story of "fly research."

Meredith Melville, NASA Public Relations, Clear Lake, Texas, supplied photos of Rhea Seddon, Patricia Santy, Shannon Lucid, and Kathryn Thornton and press releases from NASA. I conducted several interviews at the Johnson Space Center.

Canadian Elizabeth Smith's picture was provided by the University of Toronto Press with permission to publish. Photo of Dorothea Dix courtesy of Macmillan Books.

Women and Medicine is copyrighted in my name in the first edition (1980) from Scarecrow Press. In 1977, this press published *Women in Medicine: A Bibliography of the Literature on Women Physicians,* compiled and edited by Sandra L. Chaff, Ruth D. Haimbach, Carol Fenichel, and Nina B. Woodside, a work that was most helpful in my second edition published by Media Publishing (now defunct) (1988, Lincoln, Nebraska). In this third edition, the doctors themselves supplied many of the contemporary biographies.

Delores Hays Landrum drew the conceptualized portraits of Joycelyn Elders, Aletta Jacobs, Lise Meitner, Dorothy Crowfoot Hodgkin, and Christiane Nusslein-Volhard.

I am grateful to Cynthia Rothenbach for preparing the final camera-ready manuscript.

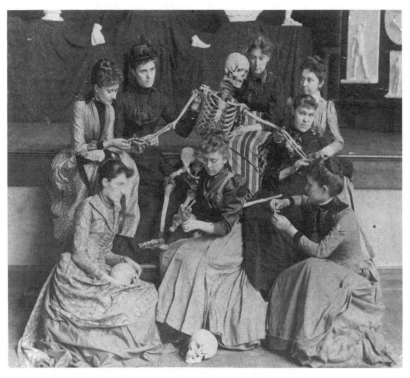

An anatomy class in 1897 at the now defunct Western College and Seminary, Oxford, Ohio. *(Photo from author's collection.)*

1

The Dinosaur Is Twitching:
Famous Firsts

In the 1970s, the American Medical Association (AMA) actively blocked the equality of women in the profession. A woman at an AMA meeting publicly pronounced the organization "prehistoric." She added, "But the dinosaur is twitching."

How far we have come! For decades, television portrayed male doctors giving orders to female nurses, technicians, and patients. Countless versions of dramas sustained the grandfather of medical myths: "The doctor is a man; trust his advice. Follow his orders!"

Some revolutionary changes in attitude have taken place. No longer is health care completely controlled by men. Women now are accepted in every field of health care.

In the 1990s, statistics revealed that women constituted 50 percent of medical school classes. Some of these students were launching second careers; some, having raised families, returned to college to fulfill dreams they had put on hold. Some minorities, who had needed convincing even to apply to medical school, did well in the most difficult courses.

Nancy Wilson Dickey

The traditionally conservative AMA, the largest organization of doctors in the United States, finally, after 150 years, changed step to elect by acclamation its first woman president. Dr. Nancy W. Dickey of College Station, Texas, ran unopposed for the one-year term in June 1997.

Dickey's colleagues praise her intelligence. "Tough as nails," they say, "an ideal person for the presidency." Dr. Dickey, a graduate of the University of Texas Medical School at Houston (Memorial Hospital System), developed indigent care programs, while directing a family practice residency in Brazos Valley, Texas. She was a professor in the department of Family and Community Medicine, College of Medicine, Texas A&M University.

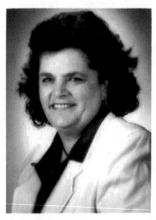

While in her forties, Dickey chaired the AMA board of trustees (a more powerful role than the presidency, though somewhat less visible). She had been a board member since 1989, excelling on the AMA Council on Ethical and Judicial Affairs. In November 1995, she was the first female board chair.

Her interest and expertise in ethics caused her to be a conscience for the AMA and for lobbying, teaching, and publishing activities that had a significant impact on medical opinion and public policy.

Widely published in medical journals and women's magazines, she addresses the subject of female roles in organized medicine.

Nancy Wilson Dickey, president of the American Medical Association, 1997. (*Photo courtesy of Nancy Wilson Dickey.*)

Dickey supports council opinions that claim it is ethical to withdraw artificial nutrition and hydration from terminally ill patients, "providing, of course, that's their desire. Or someone who is an appropriate substitute makes the request." The AMA startled the world with its first articulation of that idea in 1984.

Dickey grew up on a South Dakota farm and moved with her family to Texas when she was a teen. A counselor told her she might become a physician, but to forget it if she wanted also to be a wife and mother. Her husband, Frank Dickey, an award-winning high school sports coach, offered encouragement. "If you want to be a doctor, be a doctor."

Frances Conley

Dr. Frances Conley, writing in the prestigious medical magazine *MD* (October 1991) observed, "Unfortunately, because of the built-in hierarchical structure of the medical profession, where men are dominant and women subservient, a subtle socialization of medical practitioners begins when they are medical students and persists into and through internship and residency. The symptoms of male patients," Dr. Conley concluded, "tend to be seen as part of the disease process; whereas female patients are seen as body parts."

Stanford University hired Dr. Conley as one of only two board-certified female neurosurgeons in the United States in 1975. She drew national attention in 1991 by submitting her resignation, charging years of harassment by male colleagues in a medical school where she had been on the faculty for twenty-three years and a tenured professor of neurosurgery since 1988. Stanford created a "Task Force on Discrimination" and Conley withdrew her resignation.

However, she clung to her anger at men who have the attitude that the "whole idea that women want equality is a joke."

With her resignation, she made headlines. But it was not the first time. In the 1971 San Francisco 7.8-mile Bay to Breakers race, she was the first woman to cross the finish line, having passed 80 percent of the male runners. The newspaper the next day printed her name, marital status (married to an investment adviser who helps with cooking and shopping, Philip Conley), and a headline: "Palo Alto Housewife Wins!"

Eleanor Wallace

Against many obstacles, Dr. Eleanor Wallace became the first woman in the nation to serve as chief of medicine in a Veterans Administration hospital, overcoming the objections of the AMA to appointments of women in significant professional roles.

Changes at medical schools and in hospitals in the United States became obvious even in such a male environment as the Veterans Affairs Medical Center in Durham, North Carolina, where in 1997 a bright new clinic housed 1,400 female patients, a fellowship, and a student-training program focusing on women's health.

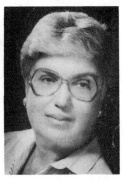

Eleanor Wallace (*Photo courtesy of Eleanor Wallace.*)

Roberta Fenlon

In 1971 newspapers in America headlined the election of Dr. Roberta Fenlon as the first women ever elected to the presidency of a state medical society. The 2,500-member California Medical Association honored Dr. Fenlon, sixty years old, a specialist in internal medicine in San Francisco and a faculty member at the University of California.

She recalled that her father opposed her ambition to become a doctor. Himself a physician, he thought medical school would be too strenuous for his daughter. Her mother urged her to be a teacher or a nurse. In the 1930s in Clinton, Iowa, Fenlon assisted her father in his medical office. Ignoring the advice of her parents, she applied to medical school when she graduated from college.

Did she encounter discrimination in medical school? "Maybe. But some of my professors also

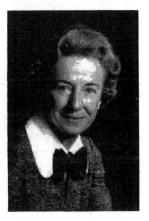

Dr. Roberta Fenlon (*Photo courtesy of California Medical Association, 1971.*)

discriminated against a few of my male colleagues. Teachers, after all, are only human."

Marcelle Willock

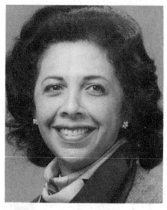

A woman committed to an academic track has to analyze whether her specialty will expose her to cutthroat competition. These women doctors are urged to teach at least one class a week.

Dr. Marcelle Willock agrees. Graduating near the top of her medical class, she had no problem getting a good surgical internship. She loved surgery but decided to switch to her second choice, a decision that led to a successful career since 1982 as chair of anesthesiology at Boston University School of Medicine.

Dr. Marcelle Willock. *(Photo courtesy of Marcelle Willock.)*

Susan Band Horwitz

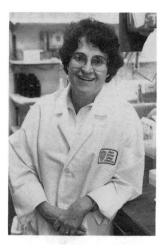

Among physicians who have been regularly promoted, Dr. Susan Band Horwitz was appointed associate director of Albert Einstein College of Medicine Cancer Research Center in Bronx, New York, in 1991. She has been associated with this prestigious institution since 1967.

She graduated from Bryn Mawr College and earned a Ph.D. degree in biochemistry at Brandeis University in 1963. Widely published, Dr. Horwitz studied taxol, a drug that may encourage antitumor activity in ovarian and breast carcinomas and malignant melanoma. Clinical trials with taxol are challenging because the drug comes from the bark of a slow-growing western yew, *taxus brevifolia*, found primarily in old growth forests in the Pacific Northwest. Removing the bark results in the death of the tree. Because some patients experience a serious allergic reaction to taxol, Dr. Horwitz is studying

Dr. Susan Band Horwitz has been widely published. *(Photo courtesy of Susan Band Horwitz.)*

semisynthetic taxol, which she hopes will help cancer patients.

Year after year since 1970, she has won honors for research, including the Outstanding Woman Scientist Award of the New York Chapter of the Association for Women in Science in 1993. She was Distinguished Lecturer in Pharmacology at St. Jude Children's Hospital as well as at Wilkes University in Wilkes-Barre, PA.

Estelle Ramey

Estelle Ramey, a biophysicist and endocrinologist who continued to lecture during her retirement after thirty-one years at Georgetown University, Washington, D.C., carried on a successful crusade with the Association of Women in Science to help "overcome the very well-known discrimination against women in salaries, promotions, and rank." She let the National Academy of Science have it.

"This is a very prestigious organization. If you get elected to it, it's helpful in the scientific community, both as to money and rank. But too few women are elected to membership."

Dr. Ramey scornfully called attention to the fact that the prestigious American Men and Women of Science had, for decades, been titled American Men of Science.

In 1929 women represented 3.5 percent of all applicants and 4.5 percent of all acceptances to medical school. The astonishingly small percentage of women doctors (before the women's movement) in the United States reflected the psychological roadblocks thrown up for girls early in life.

Medical school faculties were not always helpful. A nineteenth-century professor observed, "The only way women can be admitted here is in a pickling vat." A century later, anatomy professors still ordered students to discard breasts from female cadavers. "Stereotypes," Dr. Ramey observed, "are bred in the bone of a society. And the stereotype of the woman doctor (in the first half of the twentieth century) was of a horse-faced, flat-chested female in support hose who sublimated her sex starvation in a passionate embrace of the *New England Journal of Medicine*."

Ramey acknowledged that a young girl had to have considerable determination to ignore this threat to her image as a desirable woman. "It's enough to make a cat cry." Dr. Ramey held that "women are a remarkable and marvelous sex; the female of the species, any species, is sturdier than the male from the moment of conception to the last hurrah."

As president of the Association of Women in Science, Ramey led an organized boycott against the distribution of a medical book illustrated with seductive female nudes more suitable to a barroom calendar than to a textbook.

"Implied in the Hippocratic Oath that every doctor takes is an objective, nonprurient attitude toward patients. *The Study of Anatomy* was an obscene denigration of women and indeed of the males practicing medicine." Dr. Ramey won her crusade. The book for freshman medical students was withdrawn from the market.

Ramey, happily married to an attorney, had two children while earning a doctorate in physiology at the University of Chicago. Teaching chemistry at Queens College in New York in 1938, she became an activist for the "anonymous women in this country whose talents could move the world." In the 1980s, Ramey focused on the unprecedented health care challenge of Acquired Immune Deficiency Syndrome, AIDS. With attention paid to this devastating disease, she

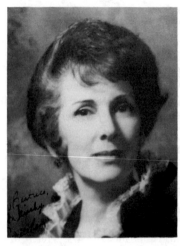

hoped that scientists studying AIDS would discover some answers to the challenges of the natural process of aging. Longer life expectancy demands finding ways to keep a graying population productive and mentally and physically fit without draining government resources.

"Aging and AIDS," Ramey noted, "attack the immune system. If we can manipulate the immune system, we can learn to affect the aging process. In terms of longevity, men are by far the weaker sex. In industrial nations, women tend to outlive men by an average of almost a decade. In brute nature, longevity was never a factor for the survival of the species. In the history of our country, more women died in childbirth than men were killed in all our wars from the French and Indian on!"

Dr. Estelle Ramey, crusader for equal pay and opportunities for women in medicine. *(Photo courtesy of Estelle Ramey.)*

Ramey admits that with the improvement in maternal health care, the scale tipped. Women's lives lengthened. Though men adopted lifestyles that included drinking, smoking, and fat-laden diets, the main reason they die sooner has to do with hormones. Testosterone causes men to react more quickly to signs of stress. Nature prepared man to fight. "Stress," she said, "may be a major culprit in increased chances of heart attacks.

"Women," Ramey concluded, "live even longer and stay healthier when men are around, perhaps because a woman prepares real meals for a man. If we can get men to live as long as women, we may reduce the cost of aging." She believes that chemical intervention may slow the body's process of aging, and anti-aging drugs may become available. For example, a study relating to the rapid aging of diabetics involved a process in which glucose, the body's blood sugar, attaches to proteins, including DNA. The experiment suggested that dietary adjustments to prevent volatile swings in glucose could slow the process of aging.

"As the public and politicians come to realize that research on AIDS may prove helpful to the aged, the nation's spending priorities might shift from weapons to health care. All that wealth," she said, "could go from death to life.

"An interesting comment on our culture," Ramey observed, "has been the number of women choosing pediatrics as a specialty. Women choose careers in child psychiatry, internal medicine, obstetrics and gynecology, and anesthesiology." However, a lasting legacy of the women's movement is that more women are becoming surgeons and entering specialties long regarded as the "masculine arena."

Jacqueline L. Wolf

Though some traditional conservative attitudes toward women physicians changed in the 1990s, Jacqueline Wolf, a greatly respected gastroenterologist and an eminently fair-minded women's liaison officer of Brigham and Women's Hospital in Boston, regrets the poor representation of women in her field. She cites statistics: In 1990, of 1,059 fellows training in this field, fewer than 12 percent were women. In 1992 in the American College of Gastroenterology, only 4 percent were women, and many often encountered sexual harassment or gender insensitivity by male colleagues. Wolf points to a survey of the Association of Women Surgeons revealing 50 percent of respondents claiming they had experienced some kind of sexual harassment or discrimination.

Are women perceived in ways different from men? Or criticized in a different way? "A man who shows anger or is aggressive is confident. A woman behaving the same way may be seen as pushy, emotional, and conceited. A man is regarded as having good judgment; a woman is said to have intuition."

Dr. Wolf believes that in academics, a glass ceiling limited the number of women on medical school faculties. In the mid-1990s, 50 percent were assistant professors, and fewer than 10 percent were full professors, compared to 31.5 percent of all men. Salary discrepancies exist in academics and practice. Though she has had remarkable recognition and regular promotions at Harvard Medical School where she teaches, she questions why women physicians, in 1988, had earned on average around 70 percent of what men earned. Even salaries in gastroenterology may not be blind to gender.

Dr. Jacqueline Wolf, associate professor at Harvard Medical School, holds the largest clinical client following at the Brigham and Women's Hospital in Boston, Massachusetts. *(Photo courtesy of Carolyn Sachs.)*

Only 2 percent of training directors in gastroenterology in 1992 were women. Only one woman was codirector in pediatric gastroenterology in 1993.

Dr. Wolf said, "Women in my specialty have too few role models and are too often taken less seriously than men. Women physicians may be more likely to pay attention to issues of abuse and the social environment that affect the patient."

Her energy and strength seem to come from her dedication to research and to her patients. She is totally convinced that doctors require not only the best possible training and education to cure illnesses and solve clinical problems but also that good medicine calls for providing guidance to improve lifestyles. Her own life has not been without anguish. In 1971, the year she left her home state of Indiana to attend Radcliffe College, her family suffered a devastating tragedy. Her younger brother, Bill, and her father, Louis Wolf, were killed in the crash of a private plane. Medicine became a consuming passion for Jacqueline, helping her to come to terms with her grief.

Married, with two daughters, Wolf exhibits a continuing enthusiasm and fascination for research projects. Among her many publications are chapters of books, reviews, editorials, reports, and abstracts. Her focus remains on patients with lacerative colitis, gastrointestinal disorders in pregnancy, and problems of bowel function.

She takes pleasure in working in her hospital and sharing companionship, ideas, and medical knowledge with other dedicated women. She was named Sandoz Scholar in Medicine in 1987. In a lecture she delivered at the Gastroenterology Training Directors' Conference in 1993, she observed, "Very few merit awards in our field go to women." She remains active in women's programs and has been the recipient of many of the highest medical awards in her field.

Rachel Fruchter

In the *New York Times* (June 22, 1997), Dr. Rachel Fruchter pointed to the way women are pursued by pharmaceutical companies as consumers. Advertisements picture radiant middle-aged women who are taking estrogen replacements and other prescription drugs.

The Health Science Center in Brooklyn concluded, "The pretense that that's what the women's health movement wanted is a bad joke. Women are now being called more frequently to a deanship or chairmanship of a medical school faculty or being elected to high office in state medical societies. No longer do we hear cliches or excuses such as 'Women are too prone to emotion, verbosity, pettiness and pregnancy.'"

Dr. Fruchter, born in London in 1949, graduated in biochemistry from Oxford University. Having earned a Ph.D. from Rockefeller University in 1966, she joined the State University of New York and pursued research that established how immigrant women without access to adequate health care suffer higher rates of cervical cancer. She also investigated how human papilloma virus relates to AIDS.

In July 1997 Dr. Fruchter, the mother of a son and a daughter, died in a bicycle accident when she swerved to avoid hitting some joggers.

To Be a Doctor in America: Overcoming Obstacles

Her inward sympathy with a doctor's and a surgeon's work grew stronger and stronger, though she dismissed reluctantly the possibility of following her bent... since, after all, her world had seemed to forbid it.

Sarah Orne Jewett, *A Country Doctor*, 1884

Deborah Crumbaker

A 1984 graduate of the University of Texas Medical School, Deborah Crumbaker had never finished high school. Nor had she earned a college degree, but she accomplished the grueling four-year obstacle course of medical school. She didn't expect it to be easy.

In Las Cruces, New Mexico, Crumbaker had always been a superior student. She would have been class valedictorian had she not had a disagreement with her parents and dropped out of school. Before submitting an application to medical school, Crumbaker had doubts about studying to be a doctor. She had worked as a nurse's aide, then in a hospital orthopedics clinic. She became familiar with casts and plasters, and had drawn excellent illustrations for a manual on tractions. Eventually she became a medical laboratory technologist. Crumbaker was thirty-two and divorced when she defied the odds by graduating from medical school. Living on a "shoestring budget" while rearing Elisa (twelve years old in 1984), Crumbaker gives her daughter credit for providing moral support. Financial assistance came from an army scholarship. After Crumbaker completed her residency, she practiced as a pathologist, a career that fulfilled her needs as a single mother. "I love medicine," she declared.

Barbara Jean Gretsch

Can a woman at age forty-five still consider starting a medical career? What if she already has eight children? And what if, in addition to raising those eight children and performing housekeeping duties, she is also employed as a district manager of the Connecticut Light and Power Company?

Certainly Barbara Jean Gretsch was not a frustrated housewife. She gave birth to two sons and five daughters in the first decade of her marriage to Richard Gretsch, an industrialist. Seven years later, a sixth daughter was born.

Barbara Jean had completed premed courses in 1942 at Transylvania University in Lexington, Kentucky, but never graduated. "At that time," she recalled, "you could do three years' pre-med and go on to medical school. It was during World War II and working my way through college, I ran out of funds."

She joined the Women's Auxiliary Army Corps and was eventually assigned to Washington, D.C. There, she met Richard Gretsch. They were married in Milwaukee in 1944. Now and then, in the years when she had only one little one at home, she would mention medical school. Her husband would murmur, "Yes, dear."

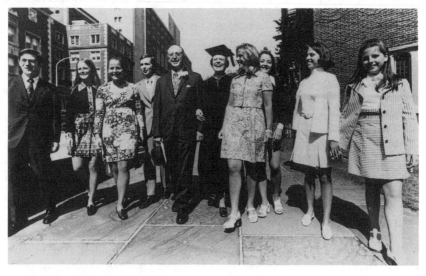

Barbara Jean Gretsch in cap and gown at her graduation from medical school, attended by her delighted family. *(Photo courtesy of Richard Gretsch.)*

Initially she applied to nearby Yale Medical School. She was told that medicine was an impossible dream for her. Perhaps she might consider studying public health? "They patted me on the head and told me to get lost," Dr. Gretsch recalled.

But at the Woman's Medical College, now the Medical College of Pennsylvania, she found a sympathetic ear. Dean Mary Hartman encouraged Gretsch, though she set tough requirements. Gretsch would have to go to an Ivy League school and repeat all the premed courses she had taken. She would have to earn straight As and achieve superior results on the Medical College Aptitude Tests.

Gretsch was eager to do all that. In the fall of 1967 at Columbia University, she began three years of study. She made the four-hour trek to class and back three days a week. In between, she gave the house a lick and a promise, prepared meals, and arranged for a babysitter for her daughter, Molly. For three years, she drove to Brewster to take the noon train and didn't return home until 1 A.M.

Against all odds, Dr. Gretsch realized her dream. "Age was my major obstacle," she claimed. For a middle-aged person, let alone a middle-aged woman, to be admitted to medical school was rare. Someone with a Ph.D. in any of the sciences and still in her thirties might be welcomed at some medical schools. While there is no set policy on age limits, and the law forbids discrimination because of sex or age, most medical schools regard someone over forty as having fewer years to practice medicine.

Dr. Gretsch's medical school classmates accepted her readily and treated her as an equal, for they were all working for the same goal. However, while they respected her dedication, they doubted she would run the strenuous course successfully.

"But some of the professors," she recalled, "would look at me and say sharply, 'Gretsch, you are old enough to know that!' "

After graduating from the Medical College of Pennsylvania in 1973, Gretsch served two years of internship and residency at St. Vincent's Hospital in Bridgeport, Connecticut.

At the age of fifty-four, Dr. Barbara Jean Gretsch, M.D., hung her shingle on Castle Hill Road and launched her family practice. She said, "I just opened the door and patients came: 3,000 in the first year and about 7,000 by 1980."

With joy and expertise, she practiced in a five-room office in the converted solarium and playroom on the main floor of her seventeen-room house in Newtown, Connecticut. The medical suite, adjacent to the kitchen, sometimes allowed patients to hear the doctor's alarm watch buzz, a reminder for someone to put supper in the oven.

Dr. Gretsch became a diplomat of the American Board of Family Practice and a fellow of the American Academy of Family Physicians. As for her remarkable achievements, she felt fortunate to be permitted to be a doctor—to do what she had always longed to do. Dr. Gretsch died suddenly in August 1980. Her courage to fulfill a dream became an inspiration to other women.

Claudia Shephard

Another atypical medical student, Claudia Shephard, was over forty when she completed residency and entered private practice. She became a doctor as a second career. A political activist at Vassar, she worked as a journalist for nine years before enrolling in Bowman Gray School of Medicine in North Carolina. "I always wanted to be a doctor when I grew up. It just took me longer to grow up. I had an undergraduate degree from Vassar in Latin. I asked myself, 'what do I look for at first when I pick up a new magazine or newspaper?' Science or medicine. I realized all my thinking was avoiding med school."

With two children, Shephard needed the moral support she received from her lawyer-husband. She continued to work full-time at the newspaper and took night classes in science. She hid her academics from colleagues. Home after 2 in the afternoon, she would relieve her babysitter and "watch her child eat small things off the rug." At 5:30, she hurried to her biology class. "I came home cross-eyed after 10:30 P.M."

Keeping this difficult schedule helped her identify and sympathize with her patients when she counseled them. She tried not to get annoyed with them. She knew what it was like to be frightened when a child is sick or to be a mother who must work while she feels rotten. "What makes me more humane is remembering how it was to live in an apartment building that burned down and having been on food stamps when my husband was unemployed. And staying up all night with a sick child."

Listening to women medical students who believe in mixing career and family, she thinks they have no idea how much distraction children are, or how tired or cross a mother gets. "In theory, you can mix a family and hard career. In practice, it's messy. The unpredictability of having children is something you don't realize before you have them. You don't realize how out of control life gets."

Leah Dickstein

Psychiatrist Leah Dickstein, associate dean for faculty and student advocacy at the University of Louisville School of Medicine in Kentucky, insisted that women must be advocates to accelerate policy changes for a systemwide adjustment. "Today," she told *MD Magazine* in April 1992, "women physicians need to be pioneers for more flexible training and practice settings, just as women in the past were pioneers for the right to enter medical school. Women who need part-time arrangements or time off to be with children need to ask for it. It is not easy for women to speak up for themselves, because they aren't accustomed to doing it, but they need to learn how."

Barbara Monstavicius

In the 1970s, Dr. Barbara Monstavicius was one of perhaps 300 women surgeons in the United States. She viewed ophthalmology as a window opening on the world, a specialty that demands meticulous attention to detail and is ideally suited to women. "I love surgery. I like the challenge. I like working with my hands."

Dr. Monstaviçius, married to a pathologist, had no children. Being an eye surgeon was a dream she cherished from childhood. Nuns who taught her in high school encouraged her. "I never expected my dream to become reality," she admitted. Practicing in San Francisco, she specialized in the use of the laser beam in eye surgery.

Dr. Monstavicius earned her medical degree at the University of Illinois, served her residency at the University of Iowa, and had a long career as a practicing surgeon. "Every time you walk into a room to see a patient or to operate, you never know exactly what the next few minutes will produce, chaos or reassurance. It's a challenge which never ends."

Dr. Monstavicius lacked enthusiasm about women electing pediatrics as their specialty. "Pediatrics, which attracts many women doctors, is a very demanding specialty. I've known women doctors whose marriages cracked up, especially if the husband wasn't in medicine. Men can't understand why wives have to get up and race out in the middle of a dinner party. Pediatricians can be overworked and overwhelmed. Many have told me this."

Leona Baumgartner

A pediatrician who became director of the Maternal and Child Health Program in New York City in 1940, Dr. Leona Baumgartner believed that women doctors deserve to have families and a career too. Data on women physicians collected since 1931 reveal that about 75 percent have married. The proportion of women doctors has increased, as has the percentage of women marrying other doctors or other medical scientists.

Susan Daum

Dr. Susan Daum, who was an internist completing residency at New York's Mt. Sinai Hospital in 1970, declared that child care should be the responsibility of society, just as health and medical treatments should be. "If the tax money now going into war and war industry could be diverted to human needs," Daum observed, "we could have all the schools, medical centers, and daycare units we wanted."

Marie Valdes-Dapena

What kind of care do we give our infants and children in the United States? A successful mother, wife, and physician, Dr. Marie Valdes-Dapena, professor of pathology at Temple University, Philadelphia, and later at the University of Miami School of Medicine, studied SIDS, sudden infant death syndrome. Performing some fifty autopsies on infants yearly, she turned her compassionate attention to parents who had lost babies.

Marie Valdes met the man she would marry while in medical school. "I had my mind set on becoming a radiologist after graduation from Temple. One day,

Antonio suggested that I apply for a residency in pathology and that we get married (not necessarily in that order)." In 1945 Marie accepted both proposals. Her husband consistently supported her career. Amazingly, Valdes-Dapena was able to carry on her successful career while having eleven children!

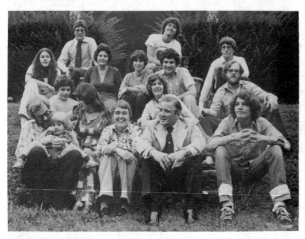

Marie Valdes-Dapena (left of center, front row) with her family, one of a series of annual family photographs of a chief pathologist associated with the University of Miami School of Nursing. She is a specialist in sudden infant death syndrome. *(Photo courtesy of Marie Valdes-Dapena.)*

Finding time for a profession and eleven children "took some doing." Fortunately, a career in pathology allowed her to leave the office behind at the end of the workday. "An important family time was supper, served at a ten-foot long table. We all ate together."

As a chief pathologist, Valdes-Dapena, with each of her six children born after 1956, worried about crib death as an unsolved medical mystery that could affect her family.

"Approximately one of every 350 infants dies suddenly, a victim of crib death," she observed. "This is one of medicine's more frightening, frustrating, unsolved mysteries. How do you convince a bereaved parent that there is no visible explanation for a child's death?" A red substance found in the baby's brain could be implicated. Death may result from parathyroid pathology, smothering, or shock, though some doctors believe a top-heavy head could cause fatal cervical injury. Valdes-Dapena suggested that the cause could be a power failure in the baby's vital mechanism that controls such functions as respiration and heart action. Perhaps low birth weight is related to crib death.

In 1990 Dr. Marie Valdes-Dapena was one of three specialists reviewing the mysterious cases of SIDS that could be either coincidence or sinister: the deaths of six babies born to a high school dropout who married three men, moved repeatedly, and tended bars. None of the babies lived longer than two years. Valdes-Dapena said, "Suffocation . . . an adult holding a hand over the baby's nose and mouth for over three minutes will kill a baby and not leave a mark." She was convinced that all the babies had been murdered. "It cannot be called SIDS if there are three or more deaths in one family," the doctor claimed.

Research on SIDS Continues

In July 2000, *The New England Journal of Medicine* reported that researchers at the University of Pavia, Italy, had provided the first genetic evidence linking SIDS to a rare heart disorder called long-QT syndrome. Doctors estimated that the heart problem could account for 25 percent of the sudden infant deaths. Many babies might be saved if all newborns were given electrocardiograms to screen for heart disorders. The infants found to have the problem could be given preventive treatment, usually drugs called beta-blockers. Most doctors recommended putting a baby to sleep on his or her back.

At the same time, doctors were telling mothers that putting a baby to sleep that way could cause the child's head to become flattened. Skull flattening may occur because a newborn has a soft, malleable skull that allows the brain to expand. The medical name is positional plagiocephaly. Most pediatricians would say, "What's that?"

In such cases it is feared that a child's head may be misshapen and ultimately require surgery. Doctors may recommend a DOC band, an expensive open-topped helmet to treat the problem. A less drastic solution is to reposition a sleeping baby's head now and then and to allow "tummy time" while the infant is awake. New mothers must be reassured that the "Back to Sleep" campaign reduced the U.S. SIDS rate by more than 40 percent from 1992 to 1998.

See also: *Trends in Pharmacological Sciences*, V. 13, p. 134 ff. April 1992

Nanette Kass Wenger

A professor of cardiology at Emory University School of Medicine, Atlanta, Georgia, Nanette Wenger was chosen Atlanta Woman of the Year in Medicine in 1972, and in 1976 was honored by *Time* magazine's Women of the Year issue for her accomplishments in cardiac rehabilitation and medical teaching. She won the American Heart Association's Award of Merit in 1978 and the Sir William Osler Award for Excellence in cardiology teaching at the University of Miami School of Medicine (Florida). In 1991 in Antwerp, Belgium, the International Association of Cardiovascular Pulmonary Rehabilitation elected Dr. Wenger as its honorary president. In 1993 she received the Vitality Award from the National Osteoporosis Foundation as well as the Women in Science President's Award from the American Medical Women's Association.

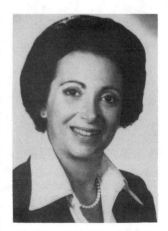

Nanette Wenger feels that studies of cardiovascular drugs for women are urgently needed. *(Photo courtesy of Nanette Kass Wenger.)*

Born in 1930, Nanette Kass Wenger graduated from Hunter College in New York in 1951. She earned her M.D. in 1954 at Harvard Medical School. Her studies of the rehabilitation of the coronary patient and cardiovascular health and disease in women have been widely published. Wenger reported that early studies showed major differences in treatment and outcome for men and women. However, by 2000, research revealed that women are as likely as men to survive heart attacks, even though they typically are treated less aggressively. One surprise in the study was that a woman was 26 percent more likely to insist on "do not resuscitate" orders stipulating that no extraordinary measure be used to prolong her life. What Wenger found encouraging was the increased attention to women who have heart attacks, the leading cause of death for both males and females. Wenger represents one woman's successful denial of the concept that women around the world are devalued as human beings.

Nancy Runge

In beautiful Estes Park, Colorado, at the Timberline Medical Clinic, the woman known as "Doctor Nancy" is a favorite with her elderly patients.

Because her grandmother was a nurse, Nancy Runge was attracted to medicine. "At first," she said, "I wanted to be a medical technologist, but I had a change in focus, inspired by a cardiologist who became my mentor. A calm, gifted physician, he taught me patience.

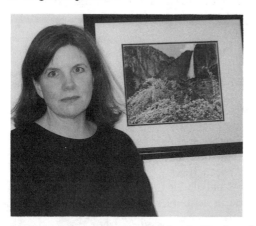

Asked to pose for a photo next to a black-and-white photo of a mountain scene, Dr. Nancy Runge gives the same close attention to the photographer as to a patient's symptoms. (*Photo from author's collection.*)

"I didn't get accepted for the first medical school where I applied. It happened to be a time when minorities were being given preference, and the prevalent attitude seemed to be the nation had enough white women doctors. I was discouraged in 1978 when Baylor University in Houston turned me down. I spent the next five years getting more competitive and those years were probably rewarding."

Did Nancy Runge make friends among the medical students? "Oh, medical school is a bonding experience. You make great friends. If you're down, there's someone to help you up." Most important are the lessons in love and the pure pleasure of pursuit of a career as a doctor.

But when she married, she learned "that medicine is a tough role to play if you don't have the support of your spouse." If a woman has a husband who is not in medicine and is jealous of the time and commitment required, the stress can be terrific.

Runge says her "comfort level is with the geriatric population. I don't birth babies, but I love watching the infants mature into children. It's fun to see how fast they change and grow up. I'm fascinated by how they learn.

"Medicine these days is hard. The business end is destroying medical care. Forty percent of our patient population are on Medicare. Fortunately, in our Timberline Medical Clinic we have contracts with groups of health associations, but we do not have restrictions imposed upon us as may be true in managed care of large populations.

"Every doctor is constantly challenged to use good judgement in what's best for the patient, in diagnosis, prescriptions, and sensible counseling.

"The summer flies, and it's a year since I had a vacation," she said. "It's an observation, not a complaint." She obviously loves being a doctor, skillfully threading a fine line between herself and her patients.

Maria Anna Scouros

Maria Scouros was born in August 1950, in Greece. She said, "I'm told I was eight years old when I first spoke of being a doctor. Early on in school in London I began taking science courses that would lead to a medical career. Being a doctor was what I wanted to do. My parents encouraged me."

Educated in London, Scouros studied internal medicine and earned a B.S. and M.S. at the Royal Free Hospital Medical School. She became a licentiate of the Royal College of Physicians. Primarily interested in understanding the cancer process and the immune system, she regarded cancer as the major medical challenge.

In 1973 she served as house surgeon at the Royal Free Hospital and in 1974 at St. Andrew's Hospital, both in London. Later in Athens, she was senior house officer at Evangelismos Hospital and at the Diagnostic and Therapeutic Center.

In 1978 she received a fellowship to study developmental therapeutics

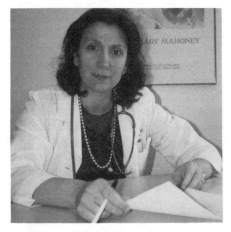

Cancer specialist Dr. Maria Anna Scouros, in private practice of oncology since 1984, directed the Center for Cancer Prevention and Treatment in Houston. (*Photo from author's collection.*)

at M.D. Anderson Hospital and Tumor Institute in Houston, Texas. She planned on two years in the United States, "but I got involved with patient care and research so I decided to stay."

Her patients may speak to her in English, Greek, Spanish, or French. She sees many patients with breast cancer. "I encourage them to do self-examinations. Patients that are at risk may have treatments of hormones. We are affiliated with NSABP, the National Surgical Adjavent Breast and Bowel Project. For patients not responding to standard treatments, we have bone marrow transplants."

She and husband, Edmond M. Haapaniemi Jr., have a daughter, born in 1989. Scouros juggles her time, her practice, and her responsibilities of home and family well.

Sally DeNardo

Dr. Sally DeNardo, at the University of California Davis School of Medicine, heads a research team studying a cancer treatment using genetically engineered molecules. This promising research has produced major shrinking of tumors in breast cancer patients who could not be helped by any other therapy. Treatment with monoclonal antibodies resulted in a 50–75 percent reduction in tumor size in six women with advanced breast cancer that had spread to other parts of their bodies.

Will this experimental approach work? The "magic bullet" technique delivers radioactive poison to tumor cells without harming the surrounding tissue. Doctors hope that this will cure the form of cancer that kills 40,000 American women every year. Physicians now believe they can prolong lives with this treatment by slowing the growth of the spreading disease and perhaps succeed where treatments such as chemotherapy and radiation have failed.

At an early stage of the experiments, Dr. DeNardo was enthusiastic. "Such clinical impact is exciting."

The good news is that applications of recombinant DNA technology work. The idea is to splice together pieces of genetic material to create new, useful combinations that do not exist in nature. Since their discovery in the mid-1970s, monoclonal antibodies have proven to be extremely complicated. At first they were used mainly to diagnose disease. Early cancer treatments had to be customized for each patient. Not every patient showed improvement. Now the treatment is moving from test tubes to the human body. Monoclonal antibodies act like guided missiles that deliver the toxin, then disappear. DeNardo's team used the new technique to deliver high doses of radioactive iodine at cancer tissue.

By attaching radioisotopes to antibodies, the therapy targets only cancer cells. According to DeNardo, "The radiation is concentrated in the tumor, stays there, and then washes out of the rest of the body. The tumor gets the medicine, and the rest of the body gets very little."

RU-486 and Breast Cancer

In 1991, America was involved in a controversy over the drug that may be helpful in treating breast cancer and other diseases affected by hormones, the abortion pill RU-486. Keeping a pill unavailable when so many women are at risk of breast cancer seemed unconscionable.

One in nine American women is at risk to develop breast cancer. In Texas, a model screening program sponsored by the state health department and other groups proved effective in encouraging women who are at risk of breast cancer to get mammograms. As part of the program, oncologists sent letters to female relatives of their breast cancer patients. The letters advised these women of their higher risk of getting cancer. A public education campaign steered women to more than 300 centers that performed mammograms for about one-third of the usual charge. Women fifty or older should have mammograms annually; those in their forties, at least every other year.

So far, unlike lung cancer (a far bigger killer caused largely by cigarette smoking), breast cancer seems to have few known avoidable causes. Epidemiologists have identified several risk factors, but fewer than half of all breast cancers have been linked to these.

A Boston oncologist, Dr. Susan Love of Harvard Medical School, regards family history as one of the most telling barometers of risk. Breast cancer seems to travel in families more than any other malignancy.

Alexandria Adler

Among the pioneer women who practiced as neurologists in the United States and Vienna, Dr. Adler studied psychological posttraumatic stress syndrome and loss of the ability to read because of brain lesions.

The daughter of the famous psychiatrist Alfred Adler, Alexandria was born in 1902 in Vienna, where she received a medical degree. She trained and practiced at the Neuropsychiatric Clinic of the University of Vienna. As editor of the *International Journal of Psychology*, she supported the branch of psychology her father pioneered after rejecting Sigmund Freud's psychoanalytical emphasis on sex as the root of neurosis.

She also interpreted Adlerian theories in a 1938 book, *Guiding Human Misfits: A Practical Application of Individual Psychology*. Several editions of the book were published in the United States, banned by the Nazis in the 1930s, and eventually republished in Germany in 1990.

After arriving in the U.S. in 1935, she taught and practiced at Harvard Medical School and Massachusetts General Hospital. In 1946 she joined the faculty at

New York University and by 1969 was full professor of psychiatry at the medical school.

Her research ranged from alcoholism to juvenile delinquency. She studied the survivors of Boston's 1942 Coconut Grove nightclub fire, one of the worst fire disasters in the United States. More than 490 people died and many of the survivors suffered brain damage. Recognizing the depression and anxiety that follow such catastrophes, she later used her research in treating traumatized World War II veterans. As a specialist in schizophrenia, Dr. Adler frequently contributed papers to reference works. At the New York City Department of Correction for two decades, she doctored female offenders. Adler also became medical director of the Alfred Adler Mental Hygiene Clinic, where she continued to study and counsel patients.

In 1959 Dr. Adler married Dr. Halfdan Gregersen, a former dean of Romance languages at Williams College. He died in 1969. Dr. Adler died January 4, 2001.

Brenda Edwards

Long involved in studying differences in survival from breast cancer between black and white women, Dr. Brenda Edwards, a biostatistician, was affiliated with the National Cancer Institute. Researching cancer prevention and control since the early days of concern about cancer, she sought answers to the effect the environment has on the disease. With her passionate interest in developing systems for cancer surveillance, she has collaborated with colleagues on quality-of-life study methodology.

Trained in biostatistics and epidemiology, Dr. Edwards, before coming to NCI, taught at a midwestern medical school and was involved in community-based and occupational studies.

Brenda Edwards, associate director, Surveillance Program, at the National Cancer Institute. (*Photo courtesy of Brenda Edwards.*)

Shirley Poduslo

In 1990 Dr. Shirley Poduslo arrived at Texas Tech Health Science Center in Lubbock to set up a DNA bank for genetic research. In two years she had organized remarkable functioning research facilities with equipment from the National Institutes of Health. The state of Texas contributed further funding. Poduslo began creating an extensive database in the community when, in 1993, she addressed a support group to families of Alzheimer patients. Among the group,

Olita Toliver, whose mother had been diagnosed with Alzheimer's disease, rallied her family to help further the research.

Poduslo explained the necessity of acquiring blood samples to help trace the flawed gene. With the community's support, by January 2000 she had collected more than 10,000 donated samples of blood and brains of deceased family members. Then her research was brought to a halt when state money earmarked for the Alzheimer project was diverted to other projects. Moreover, Dr. Poduslo was barred from her laboratory. She was ordered to destroy some 140 DNA samples because donors had not signed consent forms. Supporters of the program were disheartened at the turn of events.

"The college wants to use the money for something else," according to Maxine Cato, who had watched her mother die a terrible death from Alzheimer's in 1992. A farmer whose father had died of Alzheimer's knew that his dad's family and a number of cousins had also inherited the disease. When his father died, the farmer donated the victim's brain and blood samples to Poduslo's project. Dr. Poduslo was invited to the farmer's family reunion, where she collected more than 100 blood samples. In a few short years, three generations of the family contributed blood samples in the hope that such research would trace the flawed gene.

Until 1999, Texas state funds had been significantly specified in appropriation for the Health Science Center. That year, however, legislators freed the money from such designation. At will, university officials could allocate funds for other pursuits.

Dr. R. B. Schiffer had become chairman of the neuropsychiatry department and critical of Poduslo's work and lab techniques. He hired an outside review of her research. He may have expected a negative report, but Dr. G. M. McKahann, director of the Zanvyl Krieger Mind/Brain Institute at Johns Hopkins University wrote, "Dr. Poduslo brings to this project a strong background in neurochemistry . . . One of her great strengths is as a hands-on laboratory investigator. She has the ability to acquire new methods, refine them, and make them work." McKahann insisted Poduslo had done a remarkable job of developing the DNA bank at Texas Tech. His report was dated January 14, 2000.

Two weeks later, Poduslo was barred from her lab and her assistants were warned not to speak to her, according to a reporter, Jim Henderson, with the *Houston Chronicle* (Section 1E, February 15, 2001).

Florence P. Haseltine

Born in 1943, by the year 2000 Dr. Haseltine recalled times in medical training when male colleagues taunted or teased her: she would respond with a put-down or witticism. On occasion, she would deliver a punch or shove in response to a particularly insulting comment. She admitted she had once picked up an instructor and pitched him to the ground. Haseltine, one of seven women in her medical school class in 1970, confessed she could floor her fellow student because he

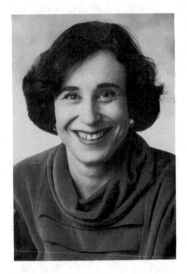

An obstetrician and gynecologist, Florence Haseltine developed a training and research program for women's health and for the professional advancement of obstetricians and gynecologists. (*Photo courtesy of Florence Haseltine.*)

was small and taken by surprise. "Women medical students had to downplay femininity . . . we learned to think like a man. My daughter is now a premedical student in a far more humane medical society. Today, in some medical schools, half the class may be women."

In 1990 Haseltine launched the Society for the Advancement of Women's Health Research and became its first president. Within three years, the society had $3 million in assets and full-time employees. Dr. Haseltine created and edited the *Journal of Women's Health* while developing Haseltine Systems, a company devoted to easing travel for the disabled.

As director of the Center for Population Research, she led a comprehensive research program in reproductive sciences and contraceptives. Specializing in reproductive endocrinology, she focused on gender differences and what they may teach us about the process of disease.

Florence Haseltine graduated from the University of California at Berkeley and holds a doctorate in biophysics from Massachusetts Institute of Technology and a medical degree from the Albert Einstein College of Medicine, Bronx, New York. She has taught in the department of ob/gyn and pediatrics at Yale and has received many honors and awards.

3

Shattering the Glass Ceiling:
Surgeons General and Presidents' Doctors

The quality of mercy is not strain'd, It drop-
peth as the gentle rain from heaven . . .
Shakespeare: *The Merchant of Venice*, Act IV,
Scene I

Surgeons General

If we define the word "grace" as to dignify and honor, we need to sing "Amazing Grace" in recognition that the United States appointed two women, a Hispanic and an African American, to protect the health of the nation.

Antonia Novello

Following in the footsteps of the remarkable Surgeon General Dr. C. Everett Koop had to be a formidable challenge for this Hispanic doctor. Koop waged war against smoking and every other threat to American health and, by the end of his eight-year tenure in 1989, was venerated by the public.

During the Senate hearing to confirm Dr. Antonia Novello, she promised to pay special attention to the health needs of women, children, and minorities. Speaking of a woman's "balancing act" and her need for help, she said, "The greatest percentage of us have children, and the greatest percentage of us have aging parents.

"My credo is: good science and good sense. In the words of Cervantes, I will not 'mince the matter.' I give you my word. I speak for those who cannot speak for themselves, particularly children. I believe that the child is, indeed, the father of the man, the mother of the woman. If you wish to take the measure of a family or a nation, you should look first at how the family or nation treats its children."

Ironically, within two years of the Senate's hearing, the United States sent mothers and fathers of infants and children to the Gulf War to risk their lives, in danger of making orphans of their offspring. Children continued to be the most disadvantaged group in America.

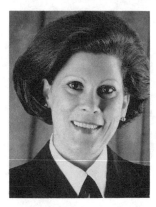

Dr. Antonia Novello, the twenty-first Surgeon General of the United States. *(Photo courtesy of Antonia Novello.)*

Dr. Novello believed that America faced an epidemic. "In cities across the nation, children are getting sick and even dying from diseases, such as measles, that are easily preventable. That is what makes this crisis particularly poignant— many of the serious childhood diseases could be completely eliminated, if only children were vaccinated on time. Today a two-year-old child in some Third World country stands a better chance of being vaccinated than a two-year-old child in inner-city America . . . one-third of our preschoolers have not been properly vaccinated against deadly diseases."

Novello regarded delaying the immunization of children until they go to school as exposing youngsters to preventable diseases such as measles, polio, mumps, and rubella. Novello created a national immunization campaign to start two-month-old babies on vaccinations and special health care programs. "Before it's too late. Vaccinate." Her crusades for early vaccination and to get young people to quit smoking probably made a greater contribution to the welfare of the youth of America than any former surgeon general had.

The appointment to the U.S. Surgeon General position stunned Novello. Well aware that in the hierarchy of medicine and politics men still run the show, she regarded her medical degree as her ultimate achievement. She had had to overcome not only prejudice against women and Hispanics in medicine, but also chronic illness.

Born in 1944 with congenital megacolon, Novello had spent part of every summer of her first eighteen years in the hospital. Novello required several corrective surgeries while she studied premed at the University of Puerto Rico. There she received an M.D. in 1970. That year, she married Joseph Novello, a naval officer and physician.

Antonia and her husband interned at Westland General Hospital, where the University of Michigan Medical School trained student physicians. Antonia had examined a patient who was later asked if she had seen a doctor. The patient replied, "Well, a Mexican nurse just came by."

Antonia, in private practice in Springfield, Virginia, once considered a career in the Public Health Service in the U. S. Navy. The captain who interviewed her said, "Didn't you hear? The U. S. Navy's looking for a few good men."

Discovering that the National Institute of Health needed kidney specialists, Novello applied. She was accepted and soon wore the uniform of a lieutenant. In 1981 she earned a master's in public health from Johns Hopkins University.

Rising rapidly through navy ranks, she headed a work group to reorganize the massive U.S. Public Health Service, chairing a task force on pediatric AIDS and cochairing a committee on women's health issues. She taught pediatrics at the Georgetown University School of Medicine. On Capitol Hill, she wrote legislative proposals, including a major law on organ donations and transplants.

In 1986, Novello was appointed deputy director of the National Institute of Child Health and Human Development. At last she seemed to have the whole world in her hand: a position that seemed to her the pinnacle of success. She had expected to continue as deputy until she retired from the Public Health Service, perhaps at age fifty-two. Then she had hoped to return to college teaching or perhaps become a dean. Never did she dream of being surgeon general.

In releasing the twenty-first surgeon general's report on smoking and health—the first issued during her tenure, she accused tobacco companies of targeting teenagers and glamorizing smoking. She herself had never smoked. "If I put a cigarette in my mouth, I thought the taste was pukey.

"Smoking continues to be the most important preventable cause of death in our society. If a person stops smoking, the risk of cancer, heart attack, stroke, and chronic lung disease is decreased. Women who stop smoking before pregnancy or during the first trimester of pregnancy reduce their risk of having a low-birth-weight baby. One in nine women is at risk to develop breast cancer, and smoking may contribute to this dread disease."

In 1991 Novello was charged with directing 5,700 commissioned public health workers hoping to educate the public about diet, smoking, nutrition, environmental health hazards, and the importance of disease prevention and immunizations. Proud of her U.S. Public Health Service uniform, she confided that she didn't like to stand up on airplanes when she was wearing it because "someone might ask me for a pillow."

"She wore her uniform well," observed her husband, Joseph Novello, a specialist in child psychiatry and a medical journalist.

As U.S. surgeon general, Dr. Novello promoted research into the health of American women. Devoted to regular aerobic exercise, she and her husband enjoyed long walks near their Georgetown home. She decorated her office with antiques and a special painting made by a child in a wheelchair. Her appetite for life and her unswerving dedication to vital traditions were revealed in her respect for this painting. "It shows that, given time and effort, you really can do wonders."

Joycelyn Elders

Joycelyn Elders, a pediatrician and an African American, considers herself a "lightning rod." Elders was in a battle most of her life, starting with her desire to escape rural Schaal, Arkansas. Enrolled in school when she was four years old, she had to walk five miles to catch a bus. At night, she helped her father stretch raccoon hides that he sold. The first in her sharecropper family of eight children to go to college, she never saw a doctor until her first year in Philander Smith, an Arkansas institution for black students. She worked her way through college as a cleaning woman. Remarkably, she graduated at eighteen!

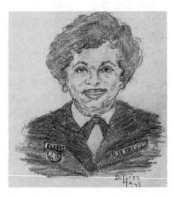

Joycelyn Elders succeeded Antonia Novello as surgeon general of the United States. *(Drawing by Delores Hays Landrum.)*

She became a first lieutenant in the U.S. Army and was trained to be a physical therapist. Imagine her loneliness later when, with the GI Bill, she was the only black woman at the University of Arkansas medical school in Little Rock. Asked by *The New York Times Magazine* reporter Claudia Dreifus if she had been an activist while in medical school, Joycelyn Elders replied, "I didn't have time for a social conscience. All I thought about was getting myself through. I didn't worry that I couldn't eat in the dining room with white students . . . I didn't worry . . . about graduation parties." Nor did she worry about people making comments about what she was doing there. A doctor told her that she had as much education "as a lot of white people." She replied, "Doctor, I have more education than most white people."

Completing a pediatric residency, she went on to earn a master of science degree in biochemistry. In 1976 she became professor of pediatrics at the Little Rock University of Arkansas Medical School, where she had felt so isolated while earning her medical degree. Dr. Elders became certified as a pediatric endocrinologist in 1978.

In 1987 Governor Bill Clinton appointed Dr. Elders as director of the Arkansas Department of Health. Under her guidance, the number of early childhood screenings in Arkansas increased from 4,000 in 1988 to 45,000 in 1992. For two-year-olds, the immunization rate increased from 34 percent in 1989 to 60 percent in 1992. Her emphasis on women receiving early prenatal care, her expanded HIV testing and counseling services, and the expansion of screenings for breast cancer won her national recognition, honorary degrees, and innumerable awards.

Time magazine, July 19, 1993, reported that the fifty-nine-year-old Arkansas public health director might have the bedside manner of a white-coat physician, but she was also a verbal bomb thrower. Striving to enlighten her home state about the health crises in teenage pregnancy and AIDS by promoting sex education, birth control, and freedom of choice on abortion, she earned many enemies.

Antiabortion activists called her a "director of the Arkansas Holocaust." Right-to-life groups challenged her nomination. She declared that abortion foes need to get over "their love affair with the fetus."*

She made headlines when she said, "If I could be the 'condom queen' and get every young person who is engaging in sex to use a condom in the United

States, I would wear a crown on my head with a condom on it! I would!" When asked if she approved of school-based clinics dispensing contraceptives, she replied, "I'm not going to place condoms on their lunch trays, but yes!"

She crusaded to convince women that the consequence of irresponsible sex is too often a child having children who grow up without proper nurturing. Elders implanted crack-addicted women with a device called Norplant that would allow them to have sex (even for pay) but not have unwanted babies.

Elders, taking up Novello's campaign to dramatize the hazards of second-hand smoke, insisted that smoking be banned in day care centers and schools. Elders hoped to influence parents of children under five living in a home with adult smokers who expose infants to acute attacks of asthma, bronchitis, and pneumonia.

Elders is not a stranger to drug problems. In 1981 she sheltered a foster child, Nina, thirteen, a blue-eyed diabetic she had been treating for five years. When Nina was twenty-five and on her own, she was arrested on a drug charge. Elders's husband paid $1,000 bail to get her out of jail. Later, Nina and her boyfriend were found murdered, perhaps because of a drug deal gone bad.

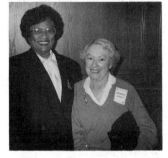

In 1993 Elders's son, Kevin, surrendered to Little Rock police to face charges of selling drugs to undercover police. The arrest came shortly after Elders suggested that legislation of

Joycelyn Elders with the author, Beatrice Levin. (*Photo from author's collection.*)

drugs merited further study and might reduce the crime rate.**

Joycelyn Elders has a sentimental side. Married since Valentine's Day, 1960, to Oliver Elders, a basketball coach at Hall High School in Little Rock until he retired, Dr. Elders rarely missed a chance to cheer at his games. Her siblings look up to their oldest sister with respect. "She cooks what mother cooked: fried chicken, turnip greens, and corn bread."

**The New York Times Magazine*, Jan. 30, 1944
**Newsweek, Feb. 14, 1994, p. 17

Presidents' Physicians

"We are not without very grave objections to women taking on themselves the heavy duties and responsibilities of the practice of medicine . . . Man, with his robust frame and trained self-command, is often barely equal to the task" was part of a resolution issued in 1867 by the Philadelphia County Medical Society.

There is no telling how many capable doctors have been lost to science be-cause women were discouraged from studying medicine.

Had Willa Cather, the famed novelist, had her wish, she would have been a doctor. Born in the home of her grandmother in Virginia in 1873, young Willa grew up fascinated by the instruments left behind by an uncle who had died shortly after he became a doctor. Young Willa studied his medical books, and in school her favorite subjects were the sciences, especially zoology. Chosen to give her high school commencement address, she spoke on "Superstition versus Investigations." She said, "It's the most sacred right of man to investigate. We paid dearly for it in Eden." She was delighted when people nicknamed her "Dr. Will."

Cather's contribution to American literature is considerable, but who knows what contribution she might have made to life sciences had she been given the slightest encouragement. Within a century, however, other determined women earned medical degrees, and two women received appointments to the White House: Dr. Ann Easton Lake and Dr. Janet Travell.

Ann Easton Lake

Very little is known of Dr. Lake's story. Born in 1849, she was educated in pediatrics. She and her husband converted the first floor of their Baltimore home into a free clinic for handicapped children. The Lakes turned a deaf ear to the protests of friends and relatives (who scorned her profession and called her "that damned Yankee who married Albert"). Idealistic Albert Lake eventually left his family firm to help with his wife's medical work. Together they were among the first people in America to make effective orthopedic appliances for crippled youngsters. Dr. Lake was appointed as a White House physician to minister to President Grover Cleveland's daughter, who suffered cerebral palsy. However, Dr. Lake had a stroke and her career ended before she ever reported to the White House.

Janet Travell

A woman physician who did report to the White House was Dr. Janet Travell. The phone rang in Dr. Travell's office on December 14, 1955. Senator John F. Kennedy of Massachusetts was calling. Would Dr. Travell fly to Palm Beach to spend the weekend with him and his wife? Senator Kennedy had been a patient of Dr. Travell's in her New York office earlier in December when he had been treated for a chronic back problem. Dr. Travell had seen a *New York Times* (September 22, 1955) photo of Kennedy leaning on crutches in a private audience with Pope Pius XII. To Travell, Kennedy joked, "I used the crutches then only because I couldn't kneel gracefully."

In Palm Beach, Dr. Travell learned that Kennedy was more uncomfortable than he would admit. Travell checked his shoes for the left heel lift she had earlier prescribed. His beach sandals lacked that correction. And he would walk barefoot on the beach, causing a disparity in leg length and creating with each step an abnormal seesaw motion in the sacroiliac and lumbosacral regions. That, said Dr. Travell, was a potential source of his back pain.

Dr. Travell ordered Kennedy to avoid going barefoot. Walking on sand involved heavy muscular effort. A special kind of strain is put on the back when someone walks on a surface sloped sideways, as on a beach. Such a slant makes one leg function as if it were longer than the other, tilting the sacrum and pelvis, causing pain. Dr. Travell assured the senator that he could swim in the ocean as long as the surf wasn't too rough. "It's more invigorating to swim in the ocean than in a pool," she said. "The water is alive and it moves you. It creates a helpful variety of both active and passive motion in a way that still water never does." Thereupon Senator Kennedy and Dr. Travell went straight to the beach and swam together in the ocean. This became one of Dr. Travell's most cherished memories.

Later Kennedy questioned the uncomfortable chairs around him. The rocker Dr. Travell ordered for his Senate office was his only really comfortable chair. When Dr. Travell joined Kennedy's White House staff in 1961, she provided the President with consistently good seating that reduced muscular fatigue. And the rocking chair Dr. Travell prescribed for the president became news and even a symbol of the Kennedy administration.

"When I was a little girl, I decided to be a doctor like my father because he was a magician and whatever he did was wonderful," wrote Travell in her autobiography, *Office Hours: Day and Night.*

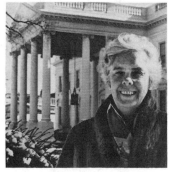

Janet Travell, President John F. Kennedy's doctor. *(Photo courtesy of Janet Travell.)*

"Through my father's eyes, every living creature became a challenging mystery. He led me to wonder, to observe, and to think about what I saw."

Janet and her sister Virginia followed their mother's example and graduated from Wellesley. Janet applied to Cornell University Medical College.

"I had witnessed the tedious hours and hard work that my father gave to his medical practice, but his unfailing enthusiasm for it was contagious." The Cornell Medical College class of 1926 graduated sixty-three students, nine of them women; Virginia's class, 1925, had contributed fifty-eight doctors, twelve of them women.

"I never had qualms about dissecting a cadaver," Janet Travell recalls. "The techniques were not strange to me after my advanced course in comparative mammalian anatomy at Wellesley."

Internship appointments were the main event in the final year at medical school. Since Travell had substituted as an intern at New York Hospital when Evelyn Holt (Wellesley, 1919)—the first woman intern in that hospital—took her vacation, Travell applied there and was accepted. At graduation, she was awarded the Polk Memorial Prize for the highest scholastic standing.

When she was twenty-five, she met Jack Powell, twenty-nine, at a dance. Janet was doing ambulance duty at New York Hospital, and Jack invited himself to sit with her. She was soon in love with him. Her uncle Sheldon, a bishop in

Chicago, agreed to come to New York to marry them in 1929 at the Church of the Ascension.

As a fellow on a clinical research project directed by Dr. Alfred E. Cohn of the Rockefeller Institute, Dr. Travell became involved in a study that combined her basic interests in pharmacology and cardiology—in science and people. In 1930 she also taught pharmacology at Cornell Medical College.

After the birth of her daughter in 1935, Dr. Travell required more flexible hours and began teaching part-time. She also continued a small private practice in her father's office. Travell considered herself fortunate for few women of that era were able to find fulfilling part-time employment.

Her father's techniques of electrotherapy were not taught in medical schools. To his office came many patients in intense pain. He used a static machine, which alerted his daughter to the crippling consequences of muscle spasms. While championing static electricity as therapy, Janet became a beneficiary of its effects. Having developed a painful right shoulder and arm, she was grateful for the periodic relief from severe pain that her father could provide with the "static surge."

Many heart-attack patients came to Janet Travell complaining about persistent pains in the shoulder region. "The Cardiac Consultation Service at Sea View," she wrote, "the city hospital for tuberculosis on Staten Island to which I was appointed in 1936, supplied the conditions that crystallized my emerging interest in muscular pain. Most patients there had life-threatening pulmonary disease, but some of them complained more about devastating pain in their shoulders and arms than about their major illness."

Dr. Travell initiated treatment of patients by local injection to the intramuscular trigger areas with procaine (Novocain). The outcome was "prompt and lasting pain relief, return of the normal range of motion at the shoulder joint, and some very grateful patients." Procaine seemed to perform miracles. A versatile drug that has been used to reduce pain in childbirth and to treat heart patients, procaine interrupts the flow of nerve impulses and may help a patient with chronic muscle spasms to find comfort. Travell was "surprised to learn that even the pain of classical myocardial infarction (i.e., heart attack) might be relieved at once by local procaine infiltration."

But among her colleagues, the therapeutic agent was subjected to bias. One colleague expressed the view that Dr. Travell could not trust her own clinical observations because she had the primary requirement for a physician—"a therapeutic personality!"

Assisted by her niece, Dr. Virginia Davidson Weeks, Travell prepared a scientific exhibit on "How to Give Painless Injections." Fear of the needle prick is an old problem in medical care. Dr. Travell remembered the limerick:

> There was a Faith Healer from Deal
> Who said, "Although pain isn't real
> When I sit on a pin
> And it punctures the skin,
> I dislike what I fancy I feel."

When Dr. Travell's two daughters started school, her husband encouraged her to continue research in heart disease and cardiac drugs at Beth Israel Hospital in New York. At the time she went to work in the White House, she was officially on leave from Beth Israel.

In the meantime, Travell spoke at medical symposiums around the world. In Galveston, Texas, in 1956, she noted the dearth of women doctors in her audience. Looking at the program, she saw that Dr. Sara M. Jordan of the Lahey Clinic was also a speaker. They met after the program to bring each other up-to-date on the medical reports of Senator Jack Kennedy. Dr. Jordan was from Boston, Dr. Travell from New York, yet it seemed natural to be discussing a mutual patient from Washington in Texas.

During his campaign for the presidency, Kennedy asked Dr. Travell to serve on the National Committee of Doctors. Sympathetic to his views on medical education, research, and care for the aged, Dr. Travell was happy to agree.

After President Kennedy's tragic death, Dr. Travell consulted with President Johnson's daughter, Luci, who years later related how she had grown up in a "can-do" family but was unable to accomplish anything scholastically significant. Tests revealed high intelligence, but Luci kept failing. "At age sixteen, I was belligerent, angry, unhappy, and frustrated. I had severe headaches and nausea." About the time her father was elected president, Luci said the source of her problems was discovered by Dr. Travell, who referred her to a Washington optometrist. Her problem was a common one: a near-point, stress-induced visual defect. Whenever she concentrated hard on anything, such as school work, she really could not see well. With proper visual correction, in less than a year Luci went from "a D-as-in-dog student to a B student."

Returning from a radiant trip to Europe in 1961 with President Kennedy and the First Lady, Dr. Travell was invited to present the commencement address at Meharry Medical College in Nashville, Tennessee. Among her remarks, she said: "No profession sets for itself such high standards of intellectual achievement and at the same time devotion to human welfare as do medicine and its partner professions. In the medical sciences, our real uniqueness lies in the fact that we often hold in our hands the specific tools for alleviating pain and illness—immediately, personally, directly. This power to relieve suffering must be nurtured with humility and never tarnished by jealousy, avarice, laziness, or disinterest on our part. It has been said that medicine is the only profession that consistently works to put itself out of business. If its goal, the conquest of disease, were achieved, what would be left for us to do?"

"The challenge of the future for medicine lies in the possibilities of modifying the behavioral patterns of the human race for the good of society."

About Abortion and Contraceptives

Volumes have been written on the pros and cons of abortion. A group of psychiatrists in 1969 recommended "abortion when performed by a licensed physician should be entirely removed from the domain of criminal law. A woman should have the right to abort or not, just as she has the right to marry or not. A patient may expect an abortion to be as routine a surgical procedure as an appendectomy." One psychiatrist insisted, "Those who oppose abortion should not avail themselves of it. A woman must have control of her own body."

Psychiatrists emphasize the moral issue on the side of abortion. "The most deadly of all possible sins is the destruction of a child's spirit," one doctor insisted. "Nothing is more harmful to a child than the conviction of being unwanted. What is more disruptive to a woman's spirit than being forced without love into motherhood? That woman, desperately seeking an abortion, poses a moral question: Should her entire life situation be threatened by an unwanted pregnancy?"

The psychiatrists were particularly critical of those opposing abortion, who made no exceptions for any reason, even rape and incest.

When society designated early abortions as murder, the courts had to deal with millions of "murders" as a legal issue that involved mass violation of the law by responsible citizens. For example in 1971, a Florida housewife, twenty-two-year-old Shirley Ann Wheeler, was warned by her doctor that her pregnancy could endanger her life because she had had rheumatic fever. Her doctor agreed to abort the fetus. When word got out, Wheeler was arrested. After a two-day trial, she admitted she had had an illegal abortion. The maximum penalty under an 1868 law was twenty years, the same as for manslaughter. Abortion supporters were so indignant and vocal that Wheeler was soon home again.

Earlier in 1967, Colorado was the first state to legalize abortion. The tradition that an abortion could be done only to save the life of the mother was abandoned. That same year, California revised the state law that had been responsible for the great number of maternal deaths due to illegal abortions. With legal abortions available, there was a dramatic reduction in the number of deaths and illnesses associated with pregnancy.

When Hawaii authorized abortion on request with a ninety-day residency requirement and other restrictions, the Hawaiian welfare system paid the bills for impoverished patients. It soon proved less expensive to help a poor woman control the size of her family than to force her to have an unwanted baby. For women who could pay for the abortion, the cost was realistic.

By 1970 New York passed an "abortion on demand" law, the most liberal in the nation, allowing an operation in the first months of pregnancy. Only the patient and her doctor were involved in the decision to abort the unwanted pregnancy. New York State nonsectarian hospitals prepared for as many as 100,000 women to come for abortions annually. Thousands, in desperation, came from other states.

In a 1973 case called *Roe v. Wade*, the U.S. Supreme Court ruled that the right to privacy protects a woman's decision to bear a child. State laws that made abortion a crime were overturned. Antiabortionists were appalled.

Since then, millions of abortions have been performed in the United States. With meticulous research, John Donohue, a law professor at Stanford University, and Steven Levitt, an economist at the University of Chicago, provided a clear benchmark against which to measure statistics that at least half the reduction of crime in the United States since *Roe v. Wade* became law is due to legalized abortion. The first states to legalize abortion were the first to experience a reduction in crime. Young women requesting abortions usually had cohorts who were at the age when a disproportionate number of crimes are committed. There was an exception in one area: more doctors who performed abortions were targeted, defamed, or murdered.

In 1998 the federal government estimated that more than 30,000 babies were abandoned in hospitals annually in the closing years of the twentieth century. In 1999 thirteen babies were found abandoned in Houston, mostly in trash bins, school yards, and alleys. Three of these infants died.

Texas Majority Whip Tom DeLay, on April 11, 2000, sponsored a bill that required state and local health agencies to track the number of abandoned infants. DeLay said, "The babies abandoned at hospitals are the lucky ones. They have instant access to health care. The little ones left in trash bins often do not live past their first day."

Of course, these are not "the lucky ones." Abandoned infants will probably never have access to a family medical history and many are traumatized.

Texas passed a landmark law excusing adults from criminal prosecution if they abandon babies at medical care facilities, a move that other states considered in the hope that desperate mothers would not be threatened with prison if they found a way to leave an infant in a safe place.

The Texas Supreme Court passed a parental notification law in 2000, signed by Governor George W. Bush, ruling that a minor girl could not have access to an abortion without first notifying her parents. One unfortunate girl feared to address her parents, since an older sister had been turned out of the home when she confessed she was pregnant. The law indiscriminately requires a teenager to go ahead with a birth she doesn't want even when the pregnancy is the result of rape or someone in her family molesting her.

Unmarried impoverished women and teenaged girls who come to clinics or doctors for abortions are sometimes the very individuals who might abandon or abuse a child or rear a potential criminal. Desperate women seeking abortion often view their very life situation as threatened.

Although white women account for the majority of abortions, blacks are three times more likely, and Hispanics twice as likely, as their white counterparts to abort a pregnancy.

Hardly a day goes by that newspapers do not carry reports of violence in schools, on the streets, and in the home. Many children raped in the home develop such low self-esteem that they become prostitutes for the rest of their lives. For such unfortunate young women, outpatient abortion is a safe procedure when performed with medical safeguards and a caring physician. Statistically, an abortion is said to be safer than a tonsillectomy and may have fewer risks than normal pregnancy and childbirth.

Throughout the world, unwanted children are permanently harmed physically and psychologically through hunger, neglect, and abuse. Some are murdered. Unwanted newborns are drowned or abandoned in dumpsters.

By 2001 a woman could plan the number and spacing of her children. She has multiple choices, including diaphragms, cervical caps, female condoms, and sponges. Occasionally, side effects from using spermicide with diaphragms and cervical caps may cause urinary tract infections. If she prefers to use birth control pills, a doctor may prescribe synthetic estrogen and progesterone. This method prevents an egg from being released by the ovaries and is said to be 99 percent effective. However, a heavy smoker is advised not to use the pill as it might increase her risk for stroke or heart attack.

A New York medical school in 1997 held a clinical trial of a contraceptive that allows a patient to have a monthly injection in her upper arm, thigh, or backside. For a busy working woman, this method proved ideal, since she usually is out of the doctor's office in fifteen minutes. When the patient decides she would like to have a child, she may expect that within two to four months of discontinuing the drug she will be pregnant.

Medically speaking, the fetus in the early months is not a person. The liver produces blood early in embryonic development, and later this task is turned over to the bone marrow. The placenta, the most vital organ in fetal metabolism, is responsible for excretion, assimilation, and respiration during pregnancy.

When the Supreme Court decreed that the mother's desires in regard to the fetus must be respected, the fetus was denied legal recognition as a human being during the first two trimesters of pregnancy. Thus the Court's ruling seemed to open the door for experiments on a fetus made available through a legal abortion. Life-threatening problems of newborn infants have long been a major area of distinguished research. The issue is terribly important: can the death of a fetus be ennobled by serving the cause of humanity, perhaps ensuring a healthy future for some much-wanted baby, or relief from suffering for someone with a disease such as Parkinson's?

4

Historical Perspectives: Midwives and Doctors around the Globe

In the fourteenth century, some women practiced as professors or doctors even if unlicensed. In Paris in 1322, Jacoba Felicie was prosecuted by the medical faculty of the University for practicing without her degree or the Chancellor's license. A witness testified that she was wiser in the art of surgery and medicine than the greatest master or doctor or surgeon in Paris. At the University of Bologna in the 1360s, the faculty included Novella d'Andrea, a woman so renowned for her beauty that she lectured behind a veil lest her students be distracted.

Barbara Tuchman, *A Distant Mirror*, p. 216

Greece

A reliable indication of how women are treated in any culture is the quality of care given women in childbirth. At the height of ancient Greek civilization, the art of caring for women in childbearing and childbirth belonged not so much to doctors as to midwives.

Most Greek gods were revered as healers, Zeus and Athena included. When the Greeks wanted a specific God of Medicine, they created out of myths and legends the wonder healer Aesculapius, an amalgam of many gods. Aesculapius was considered the son of Coronis, a maid of Thessaly, and Apollo, the sun god. Coronis may have been on her funeral pyre when Aesculapius was taken from her womb. In the myth, Aesculapius was reared by a wise old centaur who ran a one-man boarding school in a cave on Mount Pelion. Learning from a master of healing, Aesculapius surpassed his master, Cheron. From all corners of Greece, the sick and suffering came to Aesculapius, who restored their health.

35

By his first wife, Aesculapius had a daughter named Hygeia, whose name is as well-known as her father's; in its present form, we speak of hygiene, hygienic, and hygienist. Hygeia advocated preventive medicine, a concept of doctoring for healthy people as well as sick patients. Hygeia stressed "mind over matter" and used serpents to hypnotize her patients. In Greek art, Hygeia is often pictured with her father. The symbol of Aesculapius, the caduceus—two snakes entwined on a staff—survives universally as a medical emblem.

Aesculapius's second daughter, Panacea, who learned about pharmacology from her father, was devoted to all-healing herbs. Aesculapius taught her dietetic cures, surgery, and dentistry.

In the fourth century B.C., impressive temples throughout the Greek world were erected to honor Aesculapius. Adorned with art treasures and often in jewel-like settings, these temples attracted many patients. Regrettably, the priests were sometimes poor doctors. In an effort to keep a good record of patient cures ("Of course, we never lose a patient"), the priests turned away all those who were pregnant or critically ill.

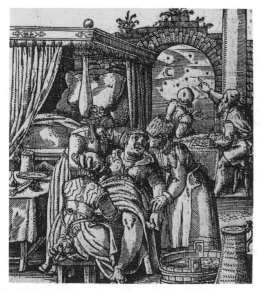

Woodcut by Jost Amman of a medieval childbirth scene. Note physicians casting horoscope and women helping with the delivery. *(Photo from author's collection.)*

At the Temple of Aesculapius, patients paid what they could afford, usually handing over an animal or a cock. Plato quotes Socrates' last words: "Crito, we owe a cock to Aesculapius; discharge this debt for me."

Aesculapius moved among the patients, touching them. The laying on of hands could achieve miraculous cures. The temples were not only hospitals, but also places of worship and Santoria, termed "Aesclepieia," which were the forerunners of our schools of medicine, hospitals, and sanatoria. Sun, fresh air, pure water, exercise, and fresh food were part of the regime. Drugs were also prescribed.

Medical instruction was oral, since there were no written medical works among the Greeks before the fifth century B.C. Completing a course in medicine, the student took an oath of Hippocrates, which in principle is as applicable today as it was to the physician 2,500 years ago: "I swear by Apollo, the physician, and Aesculapius and Hygeia and Panacea, and all the gods and all the goddesses . . . so far as power and discernment shall be mine, I will carry out a regimen for the benefit of the sick and will keep them from harm and wrong. To none will I give a deadly drug even if solicited, nor offer counsel to such end. Whatsoever in my practice or not in my practice I shall see or hear amid the lives of men, I will not divulge, as reckoning that all such things be kept secret."

In the fifth century B.C., at the time of Hippocrates, midwives were well organized. Until Emperor Antonius Pius provided a special hospital at Epidaurus for lying-in cases or for the terminally ill, midwives delivered the infant in the mother's home. Sometimes their ways with women in childbirth were crude and cruel, including kneading and rubbing the belly or forcefully lifting and dropping the patient. In extremely difficult deliveries, a doctor (called a "he-grandmother") was summoned.

Sacred songs accompanied the cries of the mother. As soon as the baby was delivered, the midwife promptly showed the infant to the father so he could acknowledge it as his own. He did this by taking the infant in his arms.

The midwife was expected to be responsible for any unwanted child. She would either leave it on a mountain or on temple steps where it would die unless some kind-hearted passerby rescued it. Childless families often watched for the midwife. Midwives were also matchmakers, providing advice on the physical eligibility of young people looking for a mate.

Ancient Greek women had no knowledge of birth control. Doctors were forbidden to perform abortions, but midwives sometimes knew how to end an unwanted pregnancy. These wise women were knowledgeable about diseases of women and were counselors as well. They were required to be past childbearing age themselves and to have had a child of their own. They cared for infants and children and often became general practitioners. We know about midwives through inscriptions on tombstones or in the works of ancient authors. Perhaps the midwives were poorly educated, since formal education was reserved for males, but some were assuredly called physicians during the period of the Republic. One such inscription speaks of Empiria, wife of Bettianus, and calls her "a woman doctor."

At the turn of the nineteenth century, in a Christian cemetery in Greece, two other names of midwives were discovered: Basila of Corycos and Thecla of Seleucia. Ancient writers, including Pliny, mention Anyte of Epidaurus; Lais of Athens; Olympias of Thebes; Salpis; Sotira; and Agnodice of Athens—probably all of them midwives.

Agnodice (around 300 B.C.) disguised herself as a man so she could specialize in women's ailments. She studied under the great physicians of her day. Discovered to be a woman, she was condemned to death. Because she had treated many noblewomen successfully, her patients came before the judges to testify they would no longer "account them for husbands or friends, but for cruel enemies that condemned Agnodice to death who had restored their health, protesting they would all die with her if Agnodice were put to death." With such an outcry and support, Agnodice was acquitted, and the law that forbade women the right to study medicine in Greece was annulled.

Agnodice was taught by Herophilus, who wrote a book to instruct midwives. Demosthenes praised the skill of women doctors and his own wife's gentle care when he was ill.

Tiraquellus points out that from the time of Agnodice, Greek women were given the rights of citizenship. He adds that even if we did not know the name of a single midwife, the fact that men were not allowed in the lying-in room except in extreme emergency indicates women must have been trained to manage labor and delivery.

At Cnidos in Asia Minor, there may have been a large group of women medical students. There, symptoms were classified in the same manner as plants. Isis and the other gods of healing were relied on to cure where human knowledge failed. Faith healing played a vital role in medicine. Theophrastus, a friend of Aristotle and inheritor of his books and garden, wrote a book of remedies, a compilation of all the teachings of the various schools around 372–287 B.C. Theophrastus classified 500 plants as Aristotle had classified animals.

Women were healers in Greece until the Golden Age ended with wars, invasions, and the Turkish occupation in the fifteenth century. Prejudice against women arrived with the Turks. Women as men's chattel became the norm until after the liberation of northern Greece in 1896, when Dr. Angelique G. Panayotatou became the first Greek woman to graduate from the Medical School of the University of Athens.

Dr. Panayotatou of Alexandria wrote a remarkable history of hygiene among ancient Greeks. Herself a descendant of a long line of Greek doctors, she wrote: "The Hellenic spirit left to all future ages its creative genius. It was the ferment of the social and intellectual organism. Its influence was never one-sided, because the Hellenic spirit never expressed itself merely by one idea but by creative acts."

Another brilliant pioneer woman doctor of Greece was Mary Kalopathakes, who went to Paris for her medical education because the University of Athens would not admit women in the early 1880s. She specialized in children's diseases, a neglected discipline in Greece at the time. Dr. Kalopathakes established nursing as a profession in Greece. She became a leader in public health work and educated the populace on the prevention of tuberculosis. In addition to writing a textbook on school hygiene courses, she edited the monthly journal *Hygeia*.

In 1902 Dr. Anthe Vassiliadou was appointed physician to the Women's Prison, where she studied the psychology of incarcerated women. At the turn of the century, Dr. Anna Katsigra, a school hygienist, refused a lectureship in obstetrics at the University of Athens because she thought she might be resented as the only woman on the staff there.

American medical women established English-speaking hospitals in Greece before America was drawn into World War I. On the Thessaloniki front, the American Unit of the Scottish Women's Hospital in Macedonia and another hospital on the Bay of Thessaloniki housed a total of 3,000 men in vast tents with "never an empty cot." These American doctors inspired their Greek counterparts to apply for admission to medical schools.

In Hippocrates' day, there were giants on the earth: Xenophon, Phidias, Socrates, Plato. Of all that have survived through history, Xanthippe is remembered as a legendary shrew who nagged Socrates to death. There was a proud band of sisters who stood at the peak of Greek civilization, who delivered babies, taught prenatal care, tended sick or healthy children, and tenderly comforted the dying. Among these unknown, unnamed women may have been some of the giants of ancient Greek medicine.

Jewish Women in Medicine

A famed midwife early in the eleventh century, Trotula, was noted for her extraordinary skills. In Salerno, Trotula had remedies for damaged maidenheads (which included putting a leech cautiously on the labia and allowing blood to trickle out to form a crust).

In the Middle Ages, despite church rulings prohibiting Jewish doctors from treating Christians, Jews dominated the medical profession, even holding high positions in the papal courts. From the twelve to the fifteenth centuries, Jewish women attended European universities and medical schools. A Jewish woman known only as Sarah, wife of Abraham, practiced and taught in Marseilles in the early 1300s.

In France, Jacoba Felicie, who may or may not have been Jewish, was fined repeatedly for practicing medicine without a license. Trained by a mentor, she was arraigned in 1322 before the Court of Justice and the Faculty of Medicine and charged with "visiting the sick in Parisian suburbs, examining urine, touching, feeling and holding their pulse, body and limbs." She explained she cared for the sick only "by God's will" and the patient's trust.

Jewish women continued to practice midwifery, although they were sometimes fined, imprisoned, and even sentenced to death if they delivered a stillborn or deformed child. Since women were exempted from military training, some were encouraged to study healing and midwifery. In Germany and Italy, the best eye doctors were women. Other women doctors had fine reputations: Rebecca Guarna, Constantia Calenda, and Francesca Romana. A Jewish woman doctor was often the wife, daughter, or widow of a doctor. In the fifteenth century, in a notorious trial, a remarkable woman doctor named Brunetta was accused of providing instruments for unproven ritual murders. Throughout the fifteenth century, Jewish women physicians were listed on the rolls of Frankfurt, Germany, and one—a Dr. Zerlin—was famous.

Aletta Jacobs

Aletta Jacobs, born in the Netherlands in 1854, was the eighth of eleven children in a Jewish family. By the time she was six years old, she had made up her mind to be a doctor. In her memoirs, Aletta recalled that her neighbors regarded her as a boy. Girls were expected to sew and bake, but Aletta preferred helping her father prepare medicines.

Despite financial hardships, the Jacobs daughters were educated in "finishing school." Aletta hated it. "Why should a girl be taught to lower her eyes if she passes a man on the street?"

When Aletta learned of a woman who had studied to become a pharmacist, she applied to the pharmacy school and received a diploma in 1870. This was a singular achievement, since higher education in Holland at that time was for men only.

Still longing to study medicine, Aletta Jacobs assisted her brother in his pharmacy. Aletta persuaded her father to write to the prime minister asking permission for her to go to Groningen University Medical School. She was qualified and received a rather reluctant acceptance for one trial year. One of her brothers, Johan, was an upper classman and declared he'd rather see her dead than in medical school. He cut her cold when they happened to be in the same room. But despite his insults and many from other male colleagues, Aletta, often ill, fulfilled all the requirements and graduated in 1878. When her father became too sick to attend to his patients, Aletta took over his practice.

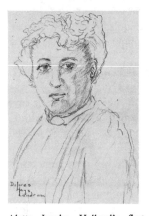

Aletta Jacobs, Holland's first woman doctor. *(Drawing by Delores Hays Landrum.)*

The Dutch press honored itself by hailing Aletta's achievements as a milestone for women. She built a strong family practice, mostly for women and children. Appalled at her patients' suffering from too-frequent pregnancies, Aletta Jacobs experimented with finding a practical contraceptive. She helped develop the diaphragm. In Amsterdam in 1878, she opened the world's first birth-control clinic. Male colleagues condemned her, charging her with causing disease of the pelvis by fitting women with diaphragms.

Dr. Jacobs defied Dutch conventions that kept decent women off Amsterdam streets during midday hours when prostitutes plied their trade. In the forefront of the women's suffrage movement, Dr. Jacobs had the support of her husband, Carol Victor Gerritsen, a radical activist who actually attended women's congresses with her. Though the Gerritsens hoped to have a family, Alleta gave birth to only one infant who lived a single day.

Dr. Jacobs survived a loving husband by twenty-four years. She devoted those years to fighting for improved working conditions for women, to peace organizations, and to birth control clinics. She died in 1929 believing "My work has succeeded. Women face a better future."

Lise Meitner

During World War I, Lise Meitner was an X-ray technician. From 1915 to 1917 Meitner was in Austrian field hospitals behind front lines. She had taken a course in roentgenology and human anatomy at City Hospital in a suburb of Berlin. Her eventual reward for her German military service, when Hitler came to power, was to be driven from her country.

Meitner was in on the discovery of uranium fission, and it was she who coined the phrase "nuclear fission." She steadfastly refused to lend her genius and creativity to developing the bomb or to any project that might lead to destruction.

She was born in 1878, the third of eight children in a Viennese family, who pronounced her name "Lee-zet" (without the "t"). She and her siblings were encouraged to study science. Her mother, a gifted pianist, taught the youngsters to play and to love music.

Lise's father believed that she should be a French teacher so she could support herself. She spent three years fulfilling his wish.

Fortunately for science, while teaching at a high school for Viennese girls, Meitner had the ambition and energy to continue her studies. With private tutors, she prepared for an examination to enter a university. In two years, she completed eight years of studies, including eight of Latin and six of Greek.

She graduated cum laude. In 1906 she was the second woman ever to receive a doctorate in physics from the University of Vienna. In 1907 Meitner went to Berlin to attend Max Planck's physics lectures. She had to use the laboratory to do her experiments when no men were present. The director of the Chemical Institute, Emil Fisher, confined her to a wood shop and barred her from other laboratories.

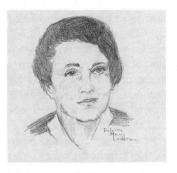

She wrote elegant articles on physics; one that was published won the admiration of the editor of *Brockhaus Encyclopedia*. He wrote "Herr Meitner" suggesting that "he" might want to write for the encyclopedia. Astonished to learn that Meitner was a woman, he rejected her prompt acceptance heatedly, saying he would not dream of publishing anything written by a woman.

Lise Meitner said, "We can no longer doubt the necessity of a woman's intellectual education." *(Drawing by Delores Hays Landrum.)*

Her part-time work with Otto Hahn was supposed to last two years, but, as Hahn records in *A Scientific Autobiography,* the years stretched to thirty "of collaboration and lasting friendship." Hahn might have been willing to share the Nobel Prize with Meitner for the discovery of nuclear fission. She did not get the recognition she deserved. Hahn listed himself as first author on their research on protactinium, though Meitner did most of the work.

Hahn and Meitner moved to the radiochemistry department of the Kaiser Wilhelm Institute for Chemistry in suburban Berlin in 1912. There, Max Planck gave her an assistantship, but it was not until the University of Prague offered her a position as an associate professor that she finally received a salary.

Shortly thereafter, Meitner became a nurse, doing X rays on wounded soldiers in an Australian army hospital. She used her leaves to work with Hahn on a search for the parent element of actinium. By 1917 she was chief of her own radiophysics department and, at last, had enough income to rent an apartment.

After World War I, when women began to be admitted to academic careers in Germany, Lise Meitner became a physics professor at the University of Berlin. In one of her first public lectures, Meitner discussed "Problems of Cosmic Physics," which a newspaper reported as "Problems of Cosmetic Physics."

Eventually, Dr. Meitner obtained not only the dignified title of German professor, but one of the proverbial attributes as well—absent-mindedness. Greeting a colleague who said, "We've already met," she replied, "You probably mistake me for Professor Otto Hahn."

When the British physicist Sir (later Lord) Ernest Rutherford met Meitner, he exclaimed, "Oh, I thought you were a man!" She was then assigned the role of hostess to his wife for the rest of Rutherford's visit.

Much respected and loved by the great physicists of her time, Meitner was known as "the gentle Lise." She had a delicious sense of humor. When Niels Bohr —whose speaking was difficult to understand—would put on one of his skits parodying famous physicists, Meitner laughed with the rest of her friends. At parties, Lise was as willing to have fun as others and danced around wearing a paper hat.

Lise Meitner became one of the great humanitarians of her age, devoting her time to helping women win admission to higher education. She regarded regulations that referred specifically to men as the problem and insisted that all that was needed was to replace the word "men" with "persons" in order to make the admission of women possible. That would also, she argued, give "women the possibility to acquire the right to lecture." She told the story of the great mathematician Dr. David Hilbert, in Göttingen, trying to obtain faculty permission for his talented woman assistant, Dr. Emmy Noether (1882–1935), to apply for the venia legendi that would make her a faculty member. He met such opposition that he snapped, "But gentlemen, a faculty is not a swimming pool!"

Nevertheless, Dr. Emmy Noether had to wait a long time before she became a lecturer. Because she was the first mathematician to show the significance of the ascending chain condition for "the ideal theory of a ring," modern mathematicians are familiar with the "Noetherian ring."

In 1935 Niels Bohr arranged a Rockefeller Foundation grant for Lise to leave Germany and work in Copenhagen for a year, but she was reluctant to abandon her research.

When the Nazis marched into Austria in 1938, Lise's very life was in danger. She no longer held a valid passport. Hahn, who had been so close a friend, gave her his mother's diamond ring for an emergency. She fled Germany on the verge of great discoveries of uranium fission. She loved Germany, where she had lived for thirty-one years. "The culmination of a life's work was snatched away."

During the twenty-two years she lived and worked in Sweden she visited the United States several times. She bequeathed her letters and papers to Cambridge University.

In 1959, when Lisa Meitner was over eighty, she spoke to students at Bryn Mawr College, reaffirming her conviction that women should become scientists, doctors, or aim for any career for which their talents and abilities qualified them. She urged them to bring their aspirations to fruition. "Undoubtedly," she declared, "women can see no ideal solutions to their problems. But for what human problems do ideal solutions exist?" She stressed that "we can no longer doubt the value and indeed the necessity of a woman's intellectual education for herself, her family, and for mankind."

In 1966 Meitner shared the Enrico Fermi Award with Otto Hahn and Fritz Strassmann, chosen for their contributions to the discovery of nuclear fission. She died two years later at the age of ninety.

In 1992 German physicists in Darmstadt fused two isotopes of bismuth and iron to make element 109, the heaviest known element in the universe. The physicist in charge, Peter Armbruster, said, "Lise Meitner should be honored for her fundamental work on the physical understanding of fission . . . honored as the most significant woman scientist of this century." The physicists named their element meitnerium to honor her.

Lucja Frey

A woman who graduated from the University of Warsaw Medical School in 1913 was one of the victims when Nazis rounded up all the Jews of Lvov in 1943. They were shot and buried in mass graves.

The name of Dr. Lucja Frey, a Polish medical scientist, appeared in a 1993 article in the *British Journal of Medical Biography* in an article by John C. Bennett. He wrote about her enormous contributions to neurological research that had been erroneously attributed to a white, male, Christian, German physician. Bennett was determined that credit for the work would go to Dr. Frey, the Polish medical scientist who had done the original and valuable research.

In January 2000, Todd Singer, a Tulsa, Oklahoma, judge, was searching the Internet for a gift for his wife, Dr. Kelley Singer, who collected memorabilia about women physicians. When Judge Singer learned of a four-page document that might be about one of Poland's top-ranking medical researchers, he did not hesitate to buy the wartime Nazi document. German-Jewish Holocaust survivors living in Tulsa translated the document and determined it was genuine. A Jewish-Christian dialogue group searched the Jewish genealogical website and found four Gottesmans who had immigrated from Lvov to the United States. Judge Singer located a Gottesman in Eugene, Oregon. He said Dr. Frey was not a relative, but he wanted to join the search. It was he who found a reference to Lucja Frey, a medical scientist responsible for discovering a neurological disorder that was named for her—Frey's syndrome.

That information led a coalition of Tulsans, both Christians and Jews, to a biography and a picture of Dr. Lucja Frey, Polish medical scientist. The dates in the biography matched those in the Nazi identity papers. Studying the Nazi document, Judge Singer felt "a hopeless hypnotic Holocaust melancholy." Frey's photo revealed to him "eyes, penetrating pools of unexplained pain, her stature, petite and gaunt."

Further research turned up a photo of the dignified young doctor seated in an ornately carved chair, wearing an elegant high-collared blouse and a long string of beads. Her beautiful hair frames a serene face. She seems every inch a true lady. With careful comparison of the facial features on this elegant photo to the one taken for the Nazi registration, Singer and dedicated assistants had accumulated evidence that Lucja Frey Gottesman had been a doctor, had completed significant research, and her name had been buried in archives.

Frey was born in 1889 in Lvov, married attorney Marek Mordekhal-Meir Gottesman, and had a daughter, Danuta. All three died in the Holocaust.

Martha Wollstein

In 1868 Martha Wollstein was born to German-Jewish parents. She entered the Woman's Medical College of the New York Infirmary in 1886. The college, founded twenty years earlier by Drs. Elizabeth and Emily Blackwell, had a fine reputation by the time Dr. Wollstein graduated. Interning at Babies Hospital in New York in 1890, she became a pathologist and concentrated on studies of malaria, tuberculosis, typhoid fever, and infant diarrhea. In 1907 Dr. Wollstein and Dr. Simon Flexner conducted the first polio experiments at the Rockefeller Institute. In 1908 Wollstein wrote a history of women's medical education in America. Later, her studies of meningitis led to the potent polyvalent sera. In 1930 she became a member of the American Pediatric Society, the first woman so honored, a fitting tribute to a distinguished pioneer in pediatric pathology.

Helen Hittner

Until recently, Jewish women who wanted to be doctors faced severe restrictions, both as women and as Jews. As Dr. Helen Hittner of Houston, a specialist in eye problems of children, said, "When I was accepted for medical school, I filled two slots for them, a woman and a Jew."

Coauthor of "Retinopathy of Prematurity, Current Concepts and Controversies," with Alice R. McPherson, M.D., and Frank L. Kretzer, Hittner wrote of the dread diseases that cause blindness in preterm babies.

Hittner, regarded with enormous respect in her profession, was a fellow of the American College of Surgeons and taught ophthalmology to Baylor University pediatricians.

Hittner graduated Phi Beta Kappa from Rice University in 1955 and was eventually accepted to Baylor University College of Medicine. One of three women among eighty medical students, she and another woman student were given a fat, bloated cadaver for the study of breasts. For a first anatomy class, breasts had to be a most unusual beginning. Determinedly, Helen worked away, refusing to succumb to disgust. The distress of their male classmates was so strong that the cadaver was eventually taken away from the women students.

Helen Hittner was reared in a close-knit family who was forever urging her male cousin to go to medical school. "Why was it so important for him to be a doctor and not for me? I began telling people that was what I wanted to do. In school, teachers would respond, 'O, be a nurse, Helen.' Sometimes people smiled or laughed, so I stopped telling them I was going to be a doctor. But I watched my cousin enroll in Rice, and I followed his example. When it came time to decide on a major, I took all the science courses."

Although Baylor College of Medicine had not exactly pounced on her application, Helen Hittner graduated with honors. She completed an internship in pediatrics. She comes from a family of pediatricians and feels comfortable among her role models. She went on to Harvard Medical School for studies in ophthalmology and her residency at Baylor-affiliated hospitals. With another Houston ophthalmologist, Dr. Alice R. McPherson, president of the Retina Society of America (one of the first doctors to help her), Helen Hittner has written an impressive number of publications. She likes writing and makes a hobby of reflecting on and recording her research.

Helen Hittner's patients are infants and children from all classes of society. She believes patient acceptance of women doctors in ophthalmology is excellent because of their greater hand dexterity and the concept of a mother-figure.

Denver Women

Throughout the 1890s, Jewish women in Denver, Colorado, recognized the need for a hospital for indigent consumptives who arrived daily, usually with one-way tickets. Most medical institutions and boardinghouses denied admittance to these deathly ill people. Hundreds of homeless invalids, coughing and hemorrhaging, lived in parks, alleys, and streets. The work of these women was no more charitable and valuable than that being achieved by other church women throughout the nation.

Frances Wisebart Jacobs

Denver's dry, sunny climate became famous for those seeking relief from tuberculosis. Among the first to suggest a free hospital for indigent "consumptive" victims was Frances Wisebart Jacobs. She was born in 1843 and became well-known for caring for the ill and the impoverished. Compassionately concerned with social problems, Jacobs would not pass a sufferer on the street without offering help. Sometimes she would pay for the services of a doctor. Known as a dynamo, the "Mother of Charities," she served on boards, raising funds, initially in the Jewish community. It was her idea to form a nonsectarian charity, the Ladies' Relief Society, and she served as the group's first vice president.

Jacobs proposed the creation of a Jewish Hospital Association. Ironically, when the list of incorporators was made, her name was not included.

By 1890 land had been purchased, and there were proposals to name the institution the Frances Jacobs Hospital as a memorial to a highly respected woman for her "humane and charitable work." She never lived to see the hospital built. She died in 1892 at the age of forty-nine. Over 4,000 people attended her ecumenical funeral.

In 1893 the hospital for which she had worked so hard had barely been erected when the Silver Crash caused a disastrous depression, destroying Denver's prosperity. The building remained vacant for six years. When at last it opened in 1899, with donated funds from throughout the nation, it had a new name: National Jewish Hospital for Consumptives.

Today, a portrait of Frances Jacobs is displayed in the rotunda of the Colorado capitol building in Denver. In addition, a fine bronze sculpture is the focal point for arriving patients and visitors in the hospital's Cohen Clinic. In recognition of her achievements, Frances Jacobs was posthumously inducted into the Colorado Women's Hall of Fame, and in 1994 into the National Women's Hall of Fame.

Seraphine Eppstein Pisko

A widow and philanthropist, Seraphine Eppstein Pisko was largely responsible for the creation of The Women's Pavilion, which was built to accommodate forty patients in an octagon solarium and wards. The solarium, with easily adjustable awnings, gave patients access to sun and fresh air year-round. Pisko was the only woman on the hospital's first board. Traveling throughout the country, she successfully raised huge contributions. In a 1914 letter, she wrote of speaking in Chicago "to almost a thousand women about the hospital." She became vice president of the hospital board and its actual administrator, since the president did not live in Denver. In 1925 the National Jewish board honored Pisko by renaming the Women's Pavilion the Seraphine Pisko Pavilion. She worked for the hospital until her death in 1941 at the age of eighty-one.

Fannie E. Lorber

When parents were hospitalized with tuberculosis, "TB orphans" often found themselves homeless. In 1907 Fannie E. Lorber, with a group of friends, established the Denver Sheltering Home for children of the patients at National Jewish Hospital. Women came to bathe the children and comfort them. By 1916, some thirty children were sheltered there, ranging in age from four to fourteen. Lorber later wrote that the home contributed to the health of the parents, whose worries about "the plight of their children often delayed the recovery of the parents." In 1969 a new Lorber building was opened as a cottage for children with asthma problems.

Israeli Women

The Israeli Women's Medical Association, founded in 1936 by forty women physicians in the home of Dr. Anna Jacob, launched women's vital roles in Israeli health care. Israel attracted women doctors, who came from every corner of the world, sometimes to serve short terms, sometimes to settle in the land of the Bible.

Henrietta Szold

The founder of Hadassah, one of the world's largest organizations of women sponsoring medical care, was Henrietta Szold. She was born in Baltimore in 1860 to Hungarian immigrants.

On a trip abroad in 1909, she visited Palestine and became enamored with the idea of helping to establish a Jewish homeland in Palestine. She had already been exposed to the Zionist ideal as a correspondent for the *Jewish Messenger* in New York. In 1893 she helped a Baltimore immigrant group organize Hebras Zion, possibly the first Zionist organization in America. That same year, she became an editor for the Jewish Publication Society where she was largely responsible for editing publications of English versions of Moritz Lazarus's *The Ethics of Judaism* and a revised edition of Heinrich Graetz's five-volume *History of the Jews*. She also contributed articles to the *Jewish Encyclopedia*.

At the founding convention of the Zionist Organization of America in Pittsburgh in 1918, Szold became director of education. That year, she originated the American Zionist Medical Unit, which partnered with other organizations to send health professionals and medical equipment and supplies to Palestine. After many challenging tasks requiring months of diplomatic negotiations and fund-raising, forty-five doctors, nurses, and administrators boarded a military convoy. They arrived in London, menaced by German ships. Finally they reached poverty-stricken Palestine.

Szold traveled between America and Palestine in 1920 and again in 1922 to supervise the reorganization of what came to be known as the Hadassah Medical Organization and became the first president of the Jewish Women's Organization.

Her greatest achievement was the role she played as director of Youth Aliyah, an agency that rescued Jewish children from Nazi Germany and settled them in Palestine. Hadassah expanded its role of training nurses and supported hospitals with other special social agencies and trade schools.

She lived in a house in Jerusalem next door to an Arab home that sheltered a "whole harem down to the third generation." Szold remembered Arab women visiting her time and again. She spoke with them with the aid of a two language dictionary.

To her dying day, Szold believed that health care, hospitals, and a higher standard of living would benefit the Arabs as well as the Israelis and that peace would come to the Holy Land.

All the years she spent in Israel, she yearned for America. She longed to walk streets with people who bathed more than once a season. She looked forward to being coddled by her sisters, having a hot toddy brought to her in bed, sleeping in a steam-heated room, and seeing a real tile bathroom.

Chloe Tal

Dr. Chloe Tal, an immunologist trained at the Hadassah Medical School, developed a test for the early detection of cancer. In 1971 she reported she had discovered a certain protein, which she called "T-globulin," in the blood of patients with cancer, and surprisingly in pregnant women. T-globulin could not be found in the blood of patients with most other diseases.

Testing 520 patients in different departments of the hospital, Dr. Tal found T-globulin in the blood of 356 of them. Subsequently, she determined that 350 of the 356 patients with T-globulin had verified cases of cancer, three were suspected but not verified as cancer patients, and three were pregnant. Thirteen patients who showed positive for T-globulin had not been diagnosed as having cancer. But within a year, the diagnosis of cancer was confirmed.

Dr. Tal believed that cancer causes the formation in the body of a specific antigen—a protein ordinarily not found in the body. The antigen causes the formation of an antibody, in this case, Dr. Tal's T-globulin. Pregnant women show the presence of T-globulin because the primitive cells in the placenta, from which the fetus derives nourishment, stimulate the production of T-globulin just as tumor cells do.

Dr. Chloe Tal, cancer specialist. (*Photo courtesy of* Hadassah Magazine, *1971.*)

Sophie Rabinoff

During World War I, Sophie Rabinoff joined the Hadassah Medical Group to organize a children's hospital and clinic for Jewish and Arab children. Born in Russia in 1889, Sophie came with her parents to the United States when she was a year old. As a child, she witnessed physicians caring for an accident victim. Inspired by their dedication, she determined to be a doctor. Sophie Rabinoff received a medical degree in 1913 from Woman's Medical College in Pennsylvania and served a residency in pediatrics at the New York Home for Hebrew Infants.

After several years in Palestine, she returned to New York to be health officer in the East Harlem Health District. In 1939 she launched an immunization program called a "whispering" campaign in parks, playgrounds, and wherever mothers gathered. The women were encouraged to bring children for diphtheria immunization. In congested, underprivileged Harlem, infant mortality was fifty-six out of every 1,000 during the first year of life. After four years of Dr. Rabinoff's program, the figure was reduced to thirty-five out of every 1,000. Harlem also had disgraceful records for tuberculosis, venereal diseases, and diabetes, problems that Dr. Rabinoff attacked with education. In 1952 she became a professor of public and industrial medicine at New York Medical College.

Dr. Rabinoff observed that from its founding, Israel considered a woman doctor an asset to family stability. By the sixties at Hadassah-Hebrew University Medical Center, medical scientists Chloe Tal, Elaine R. Berman, and a host of other women doctors were engaged in separate research attracting international respect.

Elaine Berman

In another laboratory, Professor Elaine R. Berman, for many years head of biochemistry research the Ophthalmology Department, worked closely with Dr. Tirza Cohen in the Department of Human Genetics. Their research focused on hereditary childhood diseases such as mental retardation, dwarfism, and eye problems. In 1959 Dr. Berman was invited to be in charge of the Ophthalmology Department.

"I knew nothing about eyes," she claims, but she became an authority on the pigment epithelium cell layer of the retina, the layer of the eye that lies behind the rods and cones. When her studies on diseases of middle age leading to blindness were published, she was contacted by an American cell biologist at the University of Oregon, Professor Lynette Feeney. They began a fruitful collaboration. In 1976 Dr. Berman, who was born in Chicago, returned to America for a sabbatical and joined Dr. Feeney in Oregon. In 1978 Dr. Feeney went to Israel to work on retinal pigment epithelium studies. The two women exchanged scientific data and supplemented each other's techniques, exploring retinitis pigmentosa and retinal detachment.

Dr. Berman, educated as a biochemist at the University of Chicago and Northwestern University, earned a Ph.D. in 1955. Her first husband was killed in an auto accident in 1947, three years after their marriage. In 1950 she married Rabbi Morton Berman, and the family settled in Israel in 1957. They had two American-born children, and a third was born in Israel. When Dr. Berman brought her golf clubs to Israel, Customs thought they were some kind of weapon and cross-examined her closely as to what she planned to do with the clubs. As yet, Israel had no golf course. When the Rothschilds built the golf course in Caesarea, Elaine Berman became the first women's champion golfer in Israel.

Florella Magora

Most anesthetists in Israel are women. Among them are three Hadassah specialists: Florella Magora, Kadari Avishag, and Mayera Glassman.

Dr. Magora began her studies in philosophy in Bucharest. Later, inspired by what she calls "Jewish idealism," she turned to medicine.

"I was not, however, under the impression that I was Florence Nightingale." The exceptional Bucharest faculty encouraged her to explore many options of medicine as a career.

"Anesthetics was not so sophisticated then. The procedures and apparatus were simpler. The treatment of pain and the power to bring a patient back to life excited me. This power was the essence of medicine to me." Many women who go into anesthetics believe that when you finish your role in surgery, you can be detached since you are not as involved with the patient as you are in other disciplines.

"The woman doctor choosing a career in anesthesia may think that she'll have fewer demands on her, that she will have definite working hours, but the anesthesiologist is part of a team most of the time. The work is demanding. But it's natural for a woman to want to bring relief from pain. The role of the anesthesiologist has appeal for women."

During Dr. Magora's sabbatical in France, she studied the neurophysiology of pain, a system similar to acupuncture in that it is an inhibitory process that blocks out some sensations, mainly sensations of pain.

Kadari Avishag

Dr. Magora introduced her colleague, Dr. Kadari Avishag, a small-featured woman with intelligent eyes: "Dr. Avishag is the experimental genius of the department."

Dr. Avishag originally specialized in obstetrics. Coming to Hadassah Hospital to work in intensive care units, her arrival in Jerusalem coincided with the Yom Kippur War. The wounded crowded into the hospital.

"I was desperately needed in surgery," she recalls. "Anesthetic expertise was required. With the tremendous bottleneck in our hospital, we even had dentists giving anesthesia. Every doctor, every specialist, worked day and night in surgery."

Dr. Avishag eventually became an anesthetist assigned to the pediatric intensive care unit. Hitherto, this had been an unexplored discipline in Israel. What makes her feel best, she confessed, is that sense of being needed. What could be more needed than helping a newborn fighting for life?

Dr. Avishag had five children. She recalled she was in the first group to take the boards for anesthesiology. "We had no forerunners to help us or clue us in on what to study. The next group to take the anesthesiology boards benefited from our experience and expertise."

She hoped to render operations safer, with few troublesome aftereffects in the infant, such as nausea, vomiting, and thirst. She reduced the risk of using anesthetics on babies and small children suffering congenital heart disease and other often fatal conditions, allowing doctors to operate or do procedures that previously they did not dare try.

Mayera Glassman

Dr. Mayera Glassman, also an anesthetist, is the daughter of a Hebrew teacher from Zimbabwe, South Africa, and a mother who was a bacteriologist. Both parents encouraged her to become a doctor. She was educated in Johannesburg.

"Originally, I was attracted to pediatrics, but I was discouraged from specializing in that area because I had never had any childhood diseases, so I had no immunity. I chose anesthesia because a friend of mine did." Her friend urged Dr. Glassman to go to Israel where there was a shortage of anesthetists.

The Glassman family were early Zionists. Mayera was magnetized by Israel, where she found streets named for her mother's family, the Pines. Dr. Glassman and her husband, Emanuel, a chemical engineer, have three children.

What about the general condition of women doctors in Israel? Among those who are in charge of admissions to medical school, there is a good deal of soul-searching about equality of opportunity. Fewer women than men are accepted to Israeli's four medical schools: Haifa, Tel Aviv, Beersheba, and Hebrew University in Jerusalem. Over the years, women students have frequently dropped out.

"We are a developing country," Dr. Magora explained, "and the decision to take fewer women was not easily determined." The question of military service enters into the decision. Men are required to serve three years; women only two. Women apply when they enter or finish military service and are often more mature than the men and occasionally more qualified. The entrance exam is extremely difficult. If a woman is not accepted, she may reapply or make application to schools abroad, and often she does so successfully. Medical schools are expensive to operate, and Israel cannot afford to educate potential dropouts. Women who marry or have babies after two years of medical school are costly to the program.

Places are reserved in Israeli's medical schools for Arabs, since the Arab population also needs ethnic physicians. Of course, Jewish doctors continue to serve Arab and Druze villages, providing some of the best medical care available in the Middle East.

Women physicians fight subtle discrimination on issues of medical coverage for families because of the assumption that husbands and fathers have medical insurance. Women doctors at Hadassah Hospital wanted their children to be entitled to free medical care at what they consider "their" hospital. There was also the issue of operating pajamas being issued to male surgeons while women were expected to furnish their own.

Still, women of Hadassah Hospital have won sabbaticals and other privileges and have a sense of mission and fulfillment.

Sweden

In 1901 Swedish women doctors petitioned the king to instruct the medical board to open hospital positions to unmarried women doctors who should have the same opportunities as men for positions in railway posts, towns, cities, and special tuberculosis hospitals. The document was signed by Karolina Widestrom, Hedda Anderson, Maria Folkeson, and Alma Sudquist, connected to the Polyclinic Hospital in Stockholm. Other doctors and medical students also signed the petition. The women requested that these positions pay married or single women the same salary as men received. Since they had had equal medical education, women doctors should have the same opportunities as men. The medical superintendent of the Tuberculosis Hospital attached a statement to the petition assuring the king that women were capable of filling the open positions.

His Majesty referred the petition to the Medical Council and was informed that some positions were open that were unsuitable for unmarried women, such as state prisons where inmates might endanger women. However, prisons for women could be staffed by female doctors, while men would continue to attend to male prisoners. Women made no claims to serve in the army or navy, but they did feel qualified to teach in medical school.

Anne Lavell Sundstrom

Dr. Anne Lavell Sundstrom, visiting Florida, pointed out that all Swedish citizens are entitled to free medical care. Women routinely see doctors during their pregnancy and lying-in period. The government provides a subsistence allowance for every baby.

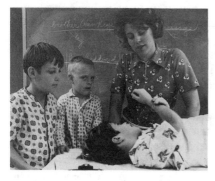

Anne Sundstrom returned to visit Florida in the 1980s. (*Photo courtesy of Florida Times-Union.*)

Dr. Sundstrom, a graduate of the Karolinska Institute in Stockholm (the college that awards the Nobel Prizes and has the largest medical school in Sweden), said that newly graduated doctors must spend three months in psychiatric practice. She served six months in general practice and the required three months in psychiatry in a remote village, making three or four house calls a day and sometimes as many as ten a day during an influenza epidemic. At the end of her long days, she would share coffee with a patient in some cottage kitchen.

As a child Sundstrom had been a gymnast. At sixteen she was stricken with polio and came to America to be treated in Florida's Hope Haven Children's Hospital. Impressed with the dedication of the doctors and what they did for her recovery, she decided to become a doctor herself.

Karolina Widerstrom

Karolina Widerstrom was the first woman to graduate from Stockholm University, the only medical school in Sweden in 1888. Of fifty to sixty graduates annually, only two or three were women. Widerstrom was born in 1856 in Halsingborg, the daughter of a veterinarian who also taught medical gymnastics. Karolina began medical studies at the Karolinska Institute in 1881. With time off for travel, she passed her finals in 1888. She practiced gynecology and taught Swedish women sex education, later publishing her lectures as a textbook, *Hygiene for Women*. She opposed a Swedish law that regulated and officially recognized prostitution as a profession. She was active on school boards and responsible for the first open-air classrooms for children with tuberculosis. A strong advocate of equal rights, she supported efforts to get women the vote and the right to hold government positions and receive equal pay. Widerstrom died in 1949.

Nanna Svartz

Nanna Svartz, born in 1890, began medical studies in 1911 in a class of sixteen men and two women. Sweden's first woman professor of medicine, Svartz specialized in children's infectious diseases, rheumatology, bacteriology, and immunology. Her gallant informal autobiography was published in Stockholm in 1968.

Alma Sudquist

Alma Sudquist, a specialist in venereal diseases and women's hygiene, gained recognition as one of the leading physicians in Stockholm. Beginning in the 1920s she worked in the Polyclinic Hospital's Department of Venereal Diseases for sixteen years. At the time, Swedish women had no organization of their own but held memberships in all the country's medical organizations. Sudquist became the fourth president of the International Association of Women.

In the mid-1940s, Sweden supported 3,600 doctors, 250 of them women. By 1960 the Swedish Medical Federation reported that 50 percent of practicing women were child psychiatrists. Three women were surgeons; one was an orthopedic specialist. There were also five gynecologists and sixteen pediatricians.

By 1994 Swedish women with aspirations to be doctors attended tuition-free medical schools. A generous welfare system provides subsidized child care and a year's paid leave after childbirth. Such assistance relieves the tension between motherhood and profession often faced by women in other countries. In 1994 women accounted for 50 percent of new Swedish Ph.D.s in fields such as molecular biology, immunology, and microbiology.

Denmark

In 1874 Nielsine Mathilde Nielsen (1850–1916) began a long struggle petitioning the Ministry of Education to admit women. When medical schools were opened to women by royal decree, Nielsine was among the first to enroll. Since Danish male physicians opposed her enrolling in a gynecology course, she went abroad to study. Her later success brought an end to that prejudice. She received her medical degree in 1885 from the University of Copenhagen, the first Danish woman to become a doctor.

She set up her practice, mostly gynecology and venereal disease, in Copenhagen in 1899. At first she faced skepticism from her patients but soon earned their respect and appreciation for her intelligence and skills. In 1906 she was appointed city venereologist. She remained active in the women's movement, struggling to get women recognition. Medicine always remained her first priority.

Finland

In 1875 Rosina Heiken became the first woman physician in Finland. Two decades were to pass before another Finnish woman graduated with an M.D. degree. For a long time, medical women faced prejudice in finding appointments to clinics. In 1994 thirty-one women physicians were practicing, bonding together in feminine comradeship and compassion. Prominent among them was psychiatrist Rakel Jalas, who became the first woman elected to the Finnish Parliament. She successfully campaigned for a law that made it possible for Finnish women to apply for state-supported maternal allowances. Dr. Jalas became a delegate to the World Health Organization and a heroine to the women of her nation.

Laimi Leidenius (1877–1938) was the first Finnish woman to receive the title of university professor of obstetrics and gynecology, in 1930. She was instrumental in planning and creating the Women's Clinic in Helsinki.

Tingvald-Hannikainen launched regular tuberculosis examinations of students at Helsinki State University in 1932. Her dedicated efforts eventually involved all schoolchildren in the Student Health Welfare Program, which became a model throughout Scandinavia in 1946.

Norway

Marie Spaangberg Holth (1865–1942) became the first Norwegian woman to graduate as a physician from the University of Norway. In 1882, the doors to medical studies were opened to women. A 1993 study revealed that Norwegian women doctors considered themselves fortunate to have better working conditions than their counterparts in many other countries. The doctors expressed pride in their work and their nation. While they were less likely to specialize than men, they enjoyed the same expanded opportunities as men in the profession. Because in the twentieth century women doctors had difficulty finding domestic and child help, many postponed marriage.

Switzerland

The University of Zurich in 1854 was the first college in the world to open its doors to women, offering complete educational equality in undergraduate and medical degrees. In the early years, only a few women studied medicine and only ten women passed the M.D. examinations. The Swiss faculty respected the dedication of the women and reported that few problems resulted from mixed classes.

Marie Heim-Vogtlin (1845–1916) was the first Swiss woman to take the same courses and examinations as male students and the first to pass the state examination. Despite poor health, she passed with distinction in 1862. She obtained her license to practice in 1873. Two years later, she married Albert Heim, a professor of geology. Blessed with a son born in 1882 and a daughter in 1886, Dr. Heim-Vogtlin began specializing in pediatrics. At the same time, she played a leading role in founding a women's hospital and a school for nurses. Eventually, she took charge of the infant care department of the new hospital. She observed the many complex problems of adoption and alcoholics. Even with a challenging regime, she never neglected her family or her home.

In 1894 American women studying at Zurich University published a guidebook for prospective students with advice on costs, behavior, course offerings, and suggestions on learning German.

The Netherlands

In 1973 E. Pereira-d'Oliverira, a family doctor and author of medical books, commemorated the fortieth anniversary of the founding of the Society of Women Physicians of the Netherlands. Her book *Women Feminists Who Practiced Medicine* traced women's emergence as doctors in the Netherlands from 1933 to their participation in World War II and postwar recovery. She discussed the problems of women doctors in marriage and child care and the offensive attitude that "a doctor is still always 'he'." Pereira-d'Oliverira cited an impressive list of papers published by women and described the founding of the Society of Women Doctors.

Belgium

What is now the Memling Museum of Brugge was formerly St. Jans Hospital. Travelers who arrived at the hospital could have a clean bed and a decent meal. Because Christians relied on God and the saints to cure illnesses, charitable hospitals became the single most valuable contribution of the medieval West.

Before a patient could be treated, a courier was required to bring a certificate ascertaining that a priest had heard confession and the invalid had received last rites. Without this religious certificate, no patient could be admitted since the infirm rarely left the hospital alive.

In the Middle Ages, treatment often involved bloodletting, even before the patient was admitted, or while hospitalized and again when leaving—that is, if the sick soul survived. Medieval doctors used herbs and drugs such as castor oil and camphor or tried to induce a kind of anesthetic by using a liquid that was mostly opium. The prevailing belief that the stars and planets influenced people's health could not have contributed greatly to curing their maladies.

The influence of medical missionaries from Belgium extended far beyond that country. A few became famous in America: Father de Smet served as the Apostle to North American Indians; Apostle Father Damien, joined by Belgian nuns, is revered for his kindness to lepers isolated on Molokai Island, Hawaii, from 1864 to 1889. Damien died of leprosy on the island; however, we are told that none of the nuns contracted the disease.

At Brugge, the nuns were cooks, laundresses, nurses, and scrub women. Other women—wives, widows, or daughters of physicians—practiced medicine. Many had passed examinations before a commission and received licenses. The Sisters at Brugge provided a precedence for Belgium's first women doctors. The first woman graduate in medicine at Brussels was Clemence Everaert (in 1803); the first at Ghent is believed to be Bertha DeVriese (in 1900).

Anne Catherine Albertine Isala van Diest (1842–1916) was born in Louvain, the daughter of a doctor. She and her five sisters and one brother all received the same education. This was most unusual for the times. After the death of the one brother, Isala was determined to be a doctor. She received a degree from the undergraduate college in Berne, Switzerland. Returning home to Louvain, she applied for admission to medical school. A sympathetic rector offered her a chance to take physiology and midwifery only. "No," she replied, "I want a medical degree." So she went back to Berne where she had made friends in college. She and twenty-two other women were admitted to study at the Faculty of Medicine. Van Diest received a medical degree in 1877 with a thesis on a South American medicinal plant. In 1882–1883 van Diest registered for courses in surgery and obstetrics. She practiced in Brussels from 1884 to 1903.

Not until 1890 did the House of Representatives in Belgium "consecrate the right of women to practice medicine and pharmacy" without discrimination against them. This reaffirmed a law of 1876 that permitted women in all the "various branches of the art of healing."

Germany

Hildegard von Bingen (1098–1178) may have been the first woman to practice medicine in Germany. During her long life, she served as abbess of Ruppetsberg Abbey. She published a number of theological and medical works, perhaps dictated in German and later translated into Latin.

Dorothea Leporin Erxleben

Dorothea Leporin Erxleben, born in 1715, and her brother were tutored in Latin, science, and the theory and practice of medicine. Around 1740, Dorothea's father and two brothers fled from Germany to evade military service. Dorothea petitioned the king and royal court to grant them pardons and allow her older brother and herself to return to their native country to study at the University at Halle. The king seems to have granted admission for the whole family. However, Dorothea's affection for a widower prompted her to give up her chance to go to the university. She married Johann Christian Erxleben, deacon of St. Nicholas in Quedlinburg. While caring for his household, she made time to write a book about education. Her supportive father wrote the foreword for her book.

Over the next dozen years, she studied medicine, wrote more books, bore four children, and provided medical care for the poor. In 1753 she became the center of a controversy when three doctors accused her of illegally practicing medicine, along with other "doctors, barbers, and midwives." Erxleben responded by requesting permission to take the doctoral examination. She passed with stunning success, the first German woman to receive a doctoral diploma. Awarded to her in 1754, it carried the signatures of the faculty and of Frederic the Great. She died of tuberculosis in 1762.

Franziska Tiburtius

Franziska Tiburtius (1843–1927), in her biography, *Memories of an Octogenarian*, recalled experiences as a medical student in Zurich, where in 1870 she was admitted to the medical school.

Upon graduation, Franziska opened a women's clinic in Berlin with a fellow medical student, Emilie Lehmus. The clinic was free. But Franziska had to have a private practice on the side to support herself. She aligned herself with other women physicians who opposed separate medical colleges for females. She held that a graduate of an exclusively female institution might be regarded as a second-class doctor. Tiburtius lived to a great old age, active and sharp to the very end.

The faculty of the University of Freiburg, as late as 1884, rejected offers for a generous endowment for scholarships for needy women in medicine and pharmacy. However, by 1895 women were allowed to audit courses. Five years later, many women were working toward a degree, and Freiburg became the first German university officially to admit women. The first gymnasium opened in Baden in 1894, followed by several others throughout Germany. At last, young women could become qualified to apply to German college degree programs in 1900.

Karen Horney

Among beneficiaries of this more liberal policy were women who became known as the "mothers of psychoanalysis:" Helen Deutsch; Melanie Klein; the daughter of Sigmund Freud, Anna; and Karen Horney. These doctors became professional psychiatrists in German-speaking Europe, and during World War II, they sought shelter in England. Eventually they settled in America.

All four psychiatrists became spokespersons for the role of psychoanalysis in the treatment of depressive, schizoid, and neurotic conditions in children and women. Challenging the views of the founder of psychoanalysis, Sigmund Freud, they called for sensitivity to the role of women, whether or not they had offspring. These doctors decried the poor quality of education for German women. Except in convent schools, most girls were trained to be middle- or upper-class wives and mothers. Music, drawing, needlework, and home economics took precedence over academic subjects. Many girls became linguists, fluent in French, Italian, English, and German.

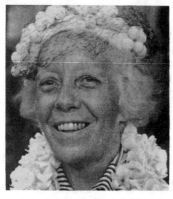

Karen Horney said, "Fortunately, analysis is not the only way to resolve inner conflicts. Life itself remains a very effective therapist." *(Photo courtesy of Brigitte Horney.)*

In the twentieth century, feminists regarded Karen Horney as a major theorist with relevance to today's woman and accepted her pioneer thinking about sexual differences. Because she herself had been in the grip of severe depression after the birth of her daughter, Horney observed how social factors play a role in common forms of maternity blues. She counseled many new mothers, some who even considered suicide. She saw mothers whose pregnancies had been difficult and observed how these women quickly became attached to their babies if they themselves had been cared for and loved.

Karen Horney, born near Hamburg, Germany, in 1885, was named Karen Clementina Theodora Danielsen. Fortunate to be educated in a fine convent school by excellent teachers, she recorded in her journals her hero-worship for her German teacher, Herr Schultz. He encouraged her ambitions, rare for a girl of that era. To please him, Karen worked diligently on his challenging assignments.

In contrast to her respect for Schultz, Karen detested her middle-class stern father, considering him a hypocrite who had expectations of others that he did not require of himself. Karen resented her parents' blatant favoritism for her older brother. Her father, a religious sea captain twenty years older than Karen's mother, Sonni, had four grown children from his first marriage. Sonni, in a loveless marriage, had two children, Berndt and Karen.

In 1906 Karen was among the first women admitted to medical school in Berlin. She passed her preclinical examinations in 1908. Karen was twenty-four when she married Oskar Horney.

Dedicated to medicine, apparently in love, and enjoying the early years of marriage, she detested housekeeping that interfered with work in the clinic. By the summer of 1910, preparing her finals, she was pregnant. Depressed by the difficulties of choosing between the socially accepted role of homemaker and the demanding role of doctor, she became even more sad when her beloved mother died of a stroke. A month later, Karen gave birth to a daughter, Brigitte.

Horney, in analysis with Dr. Karl Abraham, one of Freud's followers, was disappointed that Abraham's techniques produced few therapeutic changes. Analysis seemed only to heighten her depressions. She lost her youthful spontaneity and exuberance and substituted the semantics of analysis for her earlier, poetic prose. Despite the obvious prejudices of German professors against women doctors, Horney was permitted to take medical examinations in 1911 with a lenient examination schedule. Between tests, she cared for and nursed Brigitte. Horney's friend, Lisa Honroth, admired her dedication and offered what she regarded as a great compliment: "Karen thinks and works like a man."

During her pregnancy, Karen relished the "expectation and joy of . . . carrying in me a small becoming human being." The idea invested her with dignity and importance and made her "very happy and proud." Nursing the infant, she found an intimate union of mother and child. She longed for her own mother who had lavished loving attention on her.

Karen had had a series of affairs with men by the time she and her husband transferred to the University of Göttingen where Karen enrolled in demanding medical courses and worked in outpatient clinics. Her first patients were impoverished charity cases. Moved by the misery of these women, Karen began to reconsider the hotly controversial question of feminine sexuality. She considered that women's insecurities arose not from unflattering "spare parts" comparison with men (Freud's "penis-envy" concept) but from the cultural belittling and underevaluation of daughters.

Horney's second daughter was born in 1913 and a third in 1916. She and Oskar led an active social life, and Karen nurtured her children and continued to study philosophy and psychoanalysis. At the university, she came in contact with many women intellectually superior to men, and she observed these women's frustration over thwarted ambitions. Horney detested such bourgeois attitudes, and in rebellion, began to flirt and have affairs. However, she seems to have been ambivalent, even disturbed, about her driving need for men other than her husband and her clashing drives for independence and surrender. She hoped analysis could liberate a person who felt boxed in. She went beyond theories to introduce new concepts of human growth.

Optimistic and life-affirming, she wrote of the capacity "to wish and to will" the part of oneself that is fulfilling, the "real self." Knowing this real self, Dr. Horney believed, "leads to genuine integration and a sound sense of wholeness, oneness, and self-acceptance. The woman who finds her real self may be a better mother, a better wife, and a better human being."

In the years before World War I, the public regarded analysts as sexual perverts advocating sexual license. Horney defended her profession: "Many a marriage," she wrote, "that might have floundered because of the neurosis of one partner has become more healthy through analysis because the patient became able to direct his forces toward his marital partner, forces previously fixated on infantile models."

During World War I, she lectured on the value of psychoanalysis for social workers. She cared for many psychiatric war casualties at Lankwitz Kuranstalt. Oskar became the family disciplinarian with stern German traditions. Surprisingly, despite Karen's comprehension of childhood psychology, she managed to distance herself from Oskar's severe punishments of the girls; he beat them with a leather strap, a crop, or a stick. Karen, instead of putting a stop to this sadism, began to examine cases of women whose fears were traceable to conflicts with fathers.

The hunger and hardships of the war took their toll on the Horney family. In a hard peace, Germany was demoralized and economically devastated. During the conflict, women had operated a bus or a trolley, or worked in construction, street cleaning, or other jobs previously held by men only. Widows, now replaced by returning veterans, faced starvation and penury. Moreover, only males could enroll in college.

Dr. Horney examined her own "happy marriage" and that of others, and saw that men might consider their homes a haven, even when the wife's life was ruined and she became a drudge. She believed a man's career, when it takes precedence over his family, can have life-destroying effects.

When Oskar Horney declared financial bankruptcy, Karen may have regarded her husband as having also declared emotional bankruptcy. They were divorced.

Ironically, by 1930 Karen Horney achieved world fame as an authority on marriage. Invited with eight other German analysts to Washington, D.C., for the International Congress of Psychiatrists, she discovered life in the United States infinitely promising. She moved with her daughters to Chicago in 1932 to become the founding associate director of the Psychoanalytic Institute. She resumed the compulsive behavior with men that she had engaged in as a young woman. Known to be having affairs, she developed a long liaison with Erich Fromm. When the psychiatrist left her, Horney indignantly and vengefully tried to undermine his career. Later, feminists were furious when they learned that Horney had betrayed her patients' trust by having affairs with them.

Late in life, Karen, fascinated by Oriental religions, accepted the idea that spiritual powers develop as an individual ceases to violate an inner, true, beautiful nature. Though she has long been regarded as a leader in the early psychoanalytic movement, one of her biographers considered her work undervalued. He considered her a woman with a brilliant mind and rare talent, using her own psychic turmoil in her analytic insights. In 1932 Horney wrote "The Problem of the Monogamous Ideal," questioning why couples remain married after love is gone, a subject that may have resulted from her experiences with Oskar. Karen became an authority on why people seek extramarital affairs.

Eventually, financial rewards came to her from her readable books (most published by Norton in New York). Her insights and remarkable ability to draw from her own experiences were helpful to others. With widespread recognition, a beautiful home, and money to travel, her life became harmonious and happy. With three grown daughters, Karen Horney became convinced that women need a partner for wholeness, affection, and love.

Turkey

Anecdotal evidence supports the view that most countries have sex biases, in the way women are treated as individuals, as potential scholars, and as patients. So it comes as a pleasant surprise to learn that some Turkish women in academia have had exceptional opportunities. In the 1990s at Bosporus University, one-third of the physics and math faculty, two-thirds of the chemists, one-fifth of the engineers, and one-third of the deans were women.

A dynamic economist, Tansu Ciller left the Bosporus faculty in 1991 to become Turkey's first female prime minister. At the crossroads of Western and Islamic cultures, many women with Ph.D.s and M.D.s were thriving in exciting times.

Fellowship and research grants from the Turkish government and strong support from universities as well as an education system keeping girls on track in science support these developments. A grueling two-day exam provides the sole criterion for deciding what university they may attend and what field they will study. Ambitious high school students are tutored evenings and weekends to prepare for the exam, and girls graduate as thoroughly prepared as boys.

When the Turkish Republic was founded in 1923, the country needed educated people. Leaders sought recruits among upper-class and some middle-class women rather than among poor men, a class bias that persisted in the 1990s. With government encouragement, many women studied natural science and medicine during the last half century.

For example, Nuran Gokhan, founder of the University of Istanbul's brain research center, started medical school in 1943 in a class that was almost one-third female. She remembers there were "equal job opportunities for women in the labs." She and another woman, Meliha Terzioglu, created Turkey's first two biophysics departments at the University of Istanbul.

In the *Journal of the American Medical Women's Association* (January 1949), Perihan Cambel discussed the status of women doctors in Turkey. Recounting her meeting with Mufide Kazim (one of the first women in Turkey to study medicine), she noted that women arrived at a tea in tailor-made black suits, symbolizing their desire for dress reform. The conversation revolved around two women: Dr. Rasim Kizi Suat, among the first women physicians in Turkey, and Dr. Suat Giz, practicing surgery in a private hospital. Of the 277 women practicing medicine, most specialized in pediatrics, internal medicine, or gynecology and obstetrics. Women had to struggle for admittance to medical school and residencies. However, the women claimed there was never any discrimination against women in Turkish medical societies.

This summary obscures the fact that in the last years of the twentieth century, only 1 percent of Turkish women, a tiny minority, attained the privilege of attending college.

Only in recent years have Turkish women been emancipated. On farms, women in the fields do the heavy work. Even in the twenty-first century, Turkish country women still live in the fourteenth century, treated by men with feudal implacability. Twenty percent more females than males remain illiterate. Servants are paid a pittance.

A Turkish woman said that a man would not be caught dead doing housework. Laws about equality mean nothing. Until this changes, many Turkish women scientists and doctors choose to remain single, especially at the top ranks, where women are five times more likely than men to remain unmarried. In 1994 already 30 percent of the country's physicians were women.

Russia

Having prohibited women from pursuing a medical education in Russia, the czarist government soon found that hospitals had a severe doctor shortage in 1869. As a result, in 1872 women were urged to enroll in newly scheduled medical courses in St. Petersburg.

The first degree there was conferred on Varvara Kashevrova-Rudneva. She had studied at the Institute for Midwives in St. Petersburg in 1861 and graduated in 1862. After a year of delivering babies, she applied to the Medico-Surgical Academy, from which she graduated in 1868 with a gold medal for excellent scholarship.

When her name was called, the graduating class gave an ovation that seemed to rise to the ceiling, sending shock waves through the assembly. After her insignia was presented to her, fellow students lifted her on a chair as though she were a bride. She was carried with triumphant songs throughout the hall, while applause thundered in waves around her.

During World War II, Soviet casualties were staggering. Women were called upon to enroll in medical school. With men at the battlefront, women took over the management of hospitals and other health services.

In 2000, political attitudes toward women remained a paradox: in theory, they are "equal," but in practice, Russian women do the most menial, heavy work—ditch digging, bus driving, garbage collecting. Even where women hold professional positions, men continue to be supervisors and top managers.

Medicine as a career in Russia is not held in the high esteem it is elsewhere, and salaries are dismal. Health specialists are quick to tell you that they are not living in the best of all possible worlds. The difficulty of hiring child care or household help, the necessity of shopping on the way home from work, preparing meals, doing laundry, and keeping records may bring many women to the point of exhaustion.

Women doctors confess they sometimes accept a bribe to allow a patient to skip a waiting list and come in early. A doctor confesses she feels dishonest, but otherwise she can't make ends meet. The patient is grateful for kind attention to problems of unwanted or miserable pregnancies, birth control, childbirth, or child care. When it comes to menopause, patients particularly appreciate a sympathetic ear.

Writing in his book *Perestroika*, General Secretary Mikhail Gorbachev in 1987 observed, "We have the largest number of doctors and hospital beds per thousand of population. At the same time, there are glaring shortcomings in our health services."

Russian woman cosmonauts were expected to do medical research in space. Valentina Vladimirovna Nikolayevna-Tereshkova was the first woman in space in 1963, twenty years before the first American female astronaut, Sally Ride. In 1982 another woman cosmonaut, Svetlana Saviskaya, was launched into space. But when her Soyuz T-5 linked up with the Salyut 7 space station, the cosmonauts who had been in the space station for months greeted her with an apron, saying, "Now you can cook for us." In 1984 Saviskaya was the first Russian cosmonaut to perform a space walk.

Russian women have come a long way since the days of the czar when a popular proverb advised men: "The harder you beat the woman, the tastier the cabbage soup."

With perestroika and the failed economy, citizens of the Republic of Russia were lucky if they had even cabbage soup on the table in 2001.

Czechoslovakia

Jana Moser

When Dr. Jana Moser came to the United States in 1975, she studied as a research fellow at the Galveston Shriners Institute for Burned Children. She loved the view of the sea from the hospital windows. Moser, a plastic surgeon in the Czech Clinic of Plastic Surgery, King Charles University, regarded the Texas burn hospital as the seventh level of hell for patients. Her heart went out to children without noses, men without features, and women, who, without plastic surgery, would be condemned to a life of horror, ugliness, and pain.

As a sculptor whose art revealed beauty, grace, and form, she resolved to make living more attractive for her hospital patients. Determined not to do facelifts or fix noses for "vain women," she believed that compared to some "romantic areas of medicine, plastic surgery in burn cases is neglected. There are too few specialists, too few burn hospitals." Moser's research involved stretching the unaffected skin in burn victims to cover affected areas and using artificial skin to temporarily cover a burned area.

A homograph—grafting skin from a donor—would stay only twenty days or so. "Artificial skin works for about the same length of time," she said. The challenge, as Dr. Moser saw it, was in managing homographs. A basic treatment for burn patients has to be fluid replacement therapy. In a burn case, there is not only skin loss, but also the disruption of body organs. The burn upsets the homodynamics of the whole metabolism. The heart, blood, liver, even kidneys are affected. Most vital to survival of the patient is the percentage of body surface affected by the burn.

Dr. Moser knew that the burn victim might be deeply depressed, half out of his or her mind in shock and pain. The patient's energy must be preserved because body organs are faced with overwhelming problems—healing wounds, fighting infection, restoring metabolism, combating searing pain. "Burn hospitals require psychologists to work with burn victims," she insisted.

Olga Stastny

Having received her medical degree and acquired citizenship in the United States, Dr. Olga Stastny, a native of Czechoslovakia, became the first Czech woman to raise funds and to volunteer as a doctor for Franco-Serbian relief during World War I. In 1930 she became president of the Medical Women's National Association in the U.S. She was among the doctors at the Blackwell Medical Women's Society who spoke of the joy of working with the American Women's Hospitals serving the health needs of foreign people.

Italy

Since the Middle Ages, Italy has had a history of women who were intellectual achievers. Women were scholars from the time the first Italian universities opened during the Renaissance.

Laura Maria Caterina Bassi (1711–1778) held a chair in physics in the mid-1700s at the University of Bologna. She had a dozen children and was said to be a genius.

At the same university, Maria Dalle Donne (1778–1842) may have been the world's first woman to achieve a medical degree at the University of Bologna. Against all odds, she obtained an internship and went on to a successful practice.

Maria Montessori (1870–1952) was the first woman to earn a medical degree from the University of Rome and the first woman to care for patients in the psychiatric clinic in Rome. As a psychiatrist, she was dedicated to educating retarded children. She believed learning begins with the hands, not the brain, and she introduced exercise, rhythm games, play with toys and household utensils, and child-sized furniture. The children learned to care for little animals and plants. In 1898 she became director of a program at the University of Rome that was so successful she became convinced her methods could also be effective in teaching normal preschool children. In 1907, she opened the first *case bambini* (children's house)—a day care center. Montessori's achievements were remarkable. With devoted followers, she established schools in Europe and the United States where teachers have used her methods with generations of children in a pleasant environment. In 1933 she had to flee from Italy's fascist dictatorship. With her adopted son, she traveled to India. After the war, she returned to Europe to settle in Holland. Among many books about the Montessori method, the most interesting are those written by the remarkable founder of the educational program.

In the twenty-first century in Italy, day care is available and free for children of all working mothers. The strong Italian tradition of extended families makes reliable child care possible and gives a woman physician some freedom from worry about the welfare of her family.

In 2001, Italian girls who announced they want to study medicine were encouraged by teachers of math and science. These courses, required for all students, are taught by women who dominate high school programs, and offer hope and support to talented girls who want to be scientists, doctors, or medical researchers.

Women under the Veil

In July 1998, Taliban rulers in Kabul, the capital of Afghanistan, closed schools for girls and forced women off their jobs. Women were publicly beaten if they were not covered by the all-enveloping robe, called a burqua. European spokesman Pietro Petrucci claimed, "There is a sort of sexual apartheid. Women are being discriminated against. It violates all sorts of principles, in particular the rules of humanitarian aid."

A year earlier, fundamentalist Islamic religious police in Afghanistan had issued new regulations curbing women's access to international aid agencies operating in Kabul. Since most aid programs are directed at assisting women, especially thousands of widows, many became destitute because of laws that forbid them to work in any field except health care. Widows, according to Islamic law, should be supported by male relatives. Even in the medical sector, women had to observe certain regulations conforming to Islamic law (Sharia). No Afghan woman may take a senior or acting senior position in foreign-run hospitals. Women working in the medical sector may not sit in the seat next to the driver; no Afghan women may be transported in a car with foreigners.

Women were banned from visiting male patients in wards that contained non-family members. Makeup and jewelry were prohibited. A woman was forbidden to wear shoes with heels that might make noise when she walked in a hospital. Islamic rules that forbid a woman to work also limit her right to leave home.

Are the Taliban alone in persecuting women?

"The Egyptian woman and the Eastern woman in general suffer from a role conflict," observed Dr. Mediha el-Safty, a professor of sociology at the American University in Cairo. "On one hand, she is the modern working woman. On the other, she is still the traditional housewife with few rights."

That role model conflict was evident in spring 1997, when Fatimeh Hashemi, head of a female medical foundation with the Foreign Ministry of Iran, welcomed to her home a group of women. They arrived covered from head to foot in floor-length black "chadors" symbolizing the limited lives of Iranian women. In an elegant drawing room, they made plans for the medical foundation and the high-tech hospital Hashemi operated for kidney patients. Hashemi, the mother of two children, and daughter of Iran's president, Ali Akbar Hashemi Rafsanjani, asked the guests to summon up the courage to negotiate for change in Iran.

Hashemi and her associates, all university graduates, are among the women who make up a third of the Iranian labor force. By 1997 Iranian women had won the right to own and drive cars. They had voted in the presidential election that brought about some liberalization of harsh restrictions imposed on women by the previous fundamentalist regimes.

Women, however, were still forbidden to jog or ride a bicycle. Nor were they allowed to swim except in sexually segregated areas. They were explicitly forbidden to expose the head or neck or curve of their bodies in public. After a divorce, the father had complete control of child custody. Marriages for females were still being arranged as soon as they reached puberty. Adultery was punished by stoning to death. A women's testimony in court counted for little, always much less than a man's.

Dr. Elham Rahimian, an English-speaking radiologist, observed that most of the Iranian women coming to her for examinations were diagnosed with depression resulting from economic and psychological pressures.

In the early 1970s, when economic upheaval freed Egyptian men to travel to petroleum-producing states of the Gulf to benefit from the spectacular oil wealth, the Arab women they left behind found new independence.

Not much has changed since Dr. Hoda Badran reported in 1980, "We're now at the crossroads." At the time, Dr. Badran, a leading campaigner for women's rights and secretary-general of the National Council of Childhood and Motherhood, said that with men away, rural women for the first time handled money, hired labor to work, made family decisions, and engaged in local politics.

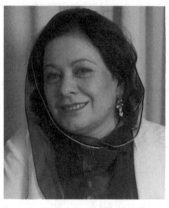

An economic decline followed, and with it a regression in social transitions. Women, now aware of the world outside their own walls, examined the rapid expansion of wealth and poverty, of personal mobility and population growth, and determined how many children they would bear, a radical change in women's attitudes.

"Men are reacting against women," Dr. Badran claimed. "If there's unemployment, it's because women are taking jobs. If there's delinquency, it's because women are leaving home to work. If there's no room on the buses, it's because women are filling them on their way to work."

Women suffer role conflicts in Moslem culture. Dr. Siddiqa Pasha keeps her head covered, even when posing for a woman photographer. *(Photo courtesy of Siddiqa Pasha.)*

Cairo newspapers headlined Egyptian wife-murders-husband stories: about Samiha who cut her spouse to pieces to dispose of his body; about Rabaa who beheaded her husband with a butcher's knife while he bowed in prayer; about Amel who stabbed her husband twenty times to avenge his brutality.

Did this mean the end or beginning of feminine liberation?

In early 1980, at the University of Tunis, Mona, a medical student, modestly made-up, wearing jeans and a colorful kerchief over her head, could be taken for a Parisian. In Saudi Arabia, Fatimeh and Waga studied at the King Faisal School of Medicine in Dammam in the department of Community and Preventive Medicine.

In Cairo, at the Medical School, women graduated as pediatricians, obstetricians, and specialists in family practice.

In Jidda, Saudi Arabia, in 1983 a new thirty-bed Siddiqa Maternity Hospital opened, staffed entirely by women. "Female patients are always more at ease detailing intimate medical complaints to a woman doctor than to a man," said Dr. Siddiqa Kamal Pasha, technical director of the new institution. "A female staff has distinct advantages in an Islamic society where women are segregated from men."

Are these then the first Arab women physicians in history? Not at all. As early as 3500 B.C. Egyptian physicians (both men and women) possessed empirical wisdom, displaying close, accurate observation. In the pharaoh's court, physicians had rank and influence. Only women doctors served the king's favorite wife and others in his harem and his royal children.

We have evidence that the nostrums of midwives were rational and useful because some were collected and recorded in papyrus rolls. What precluded progress toward real science was the trust in magic that later dominated all medical practice.

"The fertile soil of Egypt," wrote Homer, "is most rich in drugs, many of which are wholesome in solution, though many are poisonous." Egypt was famous for its drugs and poisons throughout the ancient world.

In Baghdad, women studied obstetrics in a professional school with six thousand students in the eighth century. The medical school, splendidly designed, was legendary for its sanitation and comfort. In medical schools in Cairo, Kairouan, Cordova, and Toledo, women practiced midwifery and alchemy and ministered to secluded Mohammedan women.

Alexandria, in antiquity the focal point of science and of medicine, had two celebrated royal libraries with 700,000 book rolls. Unfortunately, much of the library perished in flames around 48 B.C. when Caesar fought the Egyptians in Alexandria. When Arabs managed to rescue some books, the conquerors, eager to translate Greek scientific knowledge into Arabic, demanded that the handing-over of these texts be a condition of the peace treaty.

Arab women, some trained in medicine, translated and copied from both Latin and Greek. And in Spain, Arab libraries were impressive. The Cordova library, for example, within its first hundred years, may have acquired 200,000 volumes. Arabs coined many medical terms, such as *alcohol, naphtha,* and *camphor.* Pharmacotherapy and interest in human chemistry focused on the examination of diagnostics, so much so that there are many drawings of medieval doctors studying urine samples. The importance of pharmacology to Arab doctors became so great that it was necessary by the eighth century to separate the profession of physician from that of chemist. Most Arab medical books of the time are collections of nostrums: "Prevent him from eating anything hot," advises one doctor.

Abul Faragh, educated by Nestorians in Persia and at one time a physician to Charlemagne's family, taught midwives in the Mohammedan school in Mesopotamia. Doctor Faragh helped midwives to deliver infants in difficult births, often saving the mother's life. He was generous in his praise of the midwives' skills.

Arabs played a vital role in early studies of human anatomy. Throughout the Middle Ages, Arab armies crossed the desert, acquiring medical texts and anatomical observations from Western civilization that had been stored in Alexandria. Arab translations of these texts preserved Western scholarship, which the Christian Church at the time tried to destroy. While the Church forbade the study of human anatomy, Arab women copyists preserved the anatomical observations from early Western civilization. However, Arab religions prohibited both human dissection and pictorial representation of the human body.

Although anatomical references were limited to verbal descriptions of parts and sites of organs, Arab physicians, eager to learn about human anatomy, adapted diagrams and illustrations from Western texts. An Arab woman scholar audaciously made formal records denying the previously accepted belief that the uterus had seven parts.

Early on, women doctors in Mesopotamia studied typhoid fever, dysentery, and other diseases from infected water. Distressed by the flies that swarmed around the eyelids of children, doctors tried to teach women that flies thrived around contaminated food.

Arab women practiced in many of the sixty hospitals in Damascus when the most famous author of the ninth century, Al Rhazes (860–932), wrote the first book on pediatrics. Al Rhazes may have questioned women to help him describe measles and smallpox. He was the earliest doctor to distinguish infectious diseases characterized by rashes or skin eruptions and was surprisingly progressive for his era. He believed in the curative powers of sunlight and fresh air. Despite his wisdom, Al Rhazes ambiguously condescended to women physicians, subtitling a book "Why ignorant practitioners and common women may be more successful in curing certain complaints than better-informed physicians." He went on, "If a doctor does not cure a patient quickly, a woman doctor is called in, and she gets the credit of the cure." She also got the blame for death.

Yet elsewhere, Al Rhazes admitted he learned about herbs from women. He noted that most women doctors were content to try small doses of mild medicine rather than the massive doses recommended by their male colleagues. Some women doctors, he observed, often succeeded with tenderness and optimism. Al Rhazes, the greatest of clinicians of Islam, who died poor and blind, recorded, "Women have greater humanity than men."

Of famous Arab doctors and authors of medical books, none had a greater reputation than Avenzoar, who became the sultan's physician. Born in Seville around 1091, Avenzoar founded a great medical dynasty of Mohammedan Spain early in the twelfth century. His sons, daughter, and granddaughter were doctors. Seven generations of medical men and women carried on his work in this Mohammedan family. Tragically, his granddaughter who was a midwife and his son were both poisoned in revenge for the death of a patient.

Sir Richard Burton in *The Thousand Nights and a Night* wrote about an Arab slave girl knowledgeable about medicine, anatomy, and surgery. When medical teachers questioned her, she knew which veins to open for bleeding and what antidotes should be used for poisons. The story offers insights into what medical students learned in the Middle Ages and proves that women studied medicine.

Early Arab women doctors, unlike their male counterparts who wore silk robes, damask coats with flowing sleeves, and colorful voluminous turbans, went about with their faces veiled and bodies covered from head to foot in black robes.

A nineteenth-century Egyptian school emphasized obstetrics and distinguished between untrained midwives called "dayas" and female doctors called "hakimas" who had completed six years of training and had studied science. Six years was a long time for women who had a short life expectancy.

In 1923, an Arab woman who came to an American mission hospital for eye treatment kept asking, "Will my eyes improve in a month?" The American woman doctor, accustomed to long-suffering resignation in her patients, asked, "Why do you want to know?"

"My husband," said the patient, "gives me a month to get well. If not, he will take another wife. I'm no use to him this way."

Until recently, the Arab village that could boast a doctor was rare. The unchanging way of life led by Arabs for thousands of years is only now being affected by the scientific, medical, and educational advances of the developed world.

The first woman physician to be appointed to service of the Egyptian government, Dr. Sheldon Amos Elgood, earned an M.D. at London University in 1900. She opened the first outpatient department for women and children in an Egyptian government hospital and founded the first free children's dispensaries in Egypt. For her efforts, Dr. Elgood won the Decoration of the Nile, the Order of the British Empire, and a lasting place in the hearts of Egyptian women doctors who were able to follow in her footsteps.

Writing in 1961, Dorothy Van Ess in *Fatima and Her Sisters* observed that branding was still a favorite remedy for all kinds of sickness. Arabs, objecting to bleeding, turned to branding as treatment. A patient suffering from jaundice was advised to drink buttermilk with turmeric, then eat watermelons, and be branded on the left wrist. Stomach trouble was often treated by brandings all over the abdomen. A woman losing her eyesight as the result of corneal ulcers allowed her eyeball itself to be branded. Women doctors opposed both brandings and bleedings. Among Arab patients, curious expressions abound: an abscess is described as a "devilish wind"; the aftereffects of smallpox may be called "the cold wind of smallpox"; heart palpitation has the poetic terminology of "the flappings of a dove's wings"; a decayed tooth is "worm-eaten"; and the common cold is "the eating of a chill." Some Arabs consider a cold a month necessary to "relieve the brain" or they might go mad.

An Egyptian doctor described how Arabs tend to avoid sick people. "The value of human life is considered unimportant. Sometimes the sick are not even brought food. Inshallah, it is God's will." The last words were spoken with quiet irony.

A revolution under way behind the veils in medical education was observed by Dr. Roy G. Smith, late professor at the University of Hawaii's School of Public Health, when he was invited to teach at the King Faisal School of Medicine in Dammam, Saudi Arabia, in 1978.

The King Faisal University, founded in 1975 on the Arabic gulf, has an international faculty. Dr. Smith initiated the Comprehensive University Health

Services program for both men and women to treat indigenous diseases and health problems in response to a widespread need for community-oriented physicians in Saudi Arabia in 1978. Only 318 Saudi nationals practiced as doctors, 8 percent of the practicing physicians of the nation. Dr. Smith observed that 30 to 50 percent of Saudi medical students were female, a surprising fact in a country dominated by some of the most religiously conservative Moslem leaders in the Arab world. Men and women were totally segregated, the women taught only by women; if the lecturer were a man, closed-circuit TV was used.

Moslem culture, without eroding tradition and custom, tried to educate women physicians. Saudi women needed their husband's permission to participate in any mixed group, and then only in private homes. They were not allowed to drive. If Saudi women shopped without their husbands, custom dictated they go in pairs or trios. Outside the seclusion of walled homes, women are required to wear a black veil that covers the face and the black abaya that covers them from head to foot.

With no women on the faculty, Dr. Smith relied on classroom teaching with closed-circuit television, which created problems due to the lack of visual feedback from students. Using two-way audio, Dr. Smith required oral responses from the students. Because teaching was in English, the first year was devoted to studying English. By the second year, students could discuss issues in English, though they still had difficulty with concepts or abstractions.

To bridge the gap between the study of basic sciences and their application in actual practice, Dr. Smith assigned women students to venture into the community to deal with real patients having real problems. In such a conservative culture, the difficulties were mind-boggling. Dammam did not have a single medical clinic.

The suggestion of a house-to-house health survey captured the interest of the women students and involved them in teamwork. The first project developed a questionnaire, a survey to gather data to provide desirable learning experiences. In devising the surveys, the medical students recognized the relationship between health and environment, socioeconomic levels, health-seeking behavior, aspiration, fertility patterns, and mortality and morbidity patterns. Because of differences in class and educational levels between women students and villagers, interviewing techniques were taught with role-playing in the classroom. Women faculty members from other universities conducted face-to-face role-playing with students, at first with embarrassed giggles, but soon seriously and professionally.

The medical students feared that angry villagers would attack with sticks and stones, that the "religious police" might object, or that the army would interfere, but doomsayers' predictions did not materialize. Curious children followed the students, as Dr. Smith said, "Pied-Piper-like." Youngsters composed and sang complimentary songs about the medical students. The children were curious about strangers walking into the village without their men. They remarked about students who were taller and thinner than the village women. During the interviews, village women were responsive and friendly.

An American woman, helping the group, followed two students into a poor home. "We were welcomed," she recalled, "by an old woman swathed in black veils. Young girls and children rolled out a straw mat on the sand floor for our seats. The room was packed with visitors, many with babies, all delighted to be entertained. Questions were discussed at length in an atmosphere of good rapport. The students matured from giggling schoolgirls to future physicians."

On the second tour, a few courageous women students did not wear veils. Later, touring a hospital, they were courageous (or rebellious) enough to don blue jeans under their abayas. Students were required to wear their veils in the street or when men were present on field trips. The women knew they were under the constant surveillance of religious and military authorities. If they protested, the medical school might have been closed to them. Despite complaints from a medical student that the veil caused her asthma, she was expected to conform.

Dr. Smith recorded that during the village surveys, students distributed health education materials on nutrition and the value of immunizations and urged mothers to bring children under nine who had not been immunized to the vaccination station. The students were impressed that immunizations might prevent post-polio, paraplegic, and flaccid paralysis of a child. Dr. Smith taught students how to give immunizations, and on one occasion, the doctor created a clinical situation in which he taught the women face-to-face. This patient contact reinforced the medical students' basic concepts of preventive medicine and primary care. As the medical students began to feel more comfortable around Dr. Smith, several of them put aside their veils while examining and vaccinating babies. Many mothers of the infants also discarded their veils in the vaccination station.

Both men and women medical students presented research papers, the men on closed-circuit TV and the women on two-way audio systems. At first both sexes seemed embarrassed. The comments of the men tended to be condescending, but soon more mature attitudes developed when the men saw what formidable competitors the women were. The women, astute and aggressive in their criticism of the papers presented by the men, revealed impressive intellectual and emotional growth during the academic year. This program launched professional acceptance of women by their male peers, a development that had significant consequences for Saudi Arabian women.

"The national plan to educate women to assist in the rapid development of the country," wrote Dr. Smith, "is like opening the flood gates in a parched, arid land. The repercussions to Saudi Arabia will be as great as the industrialization plan itself."

Nawal El-Saadwi, an Egyptian doctor who wrote about Moslem culture, observed that a feeling of anger is natural among suppressed women. Marital law has not kept up with modern realities, when marriages are still arranged by relatives. Men have a legal right to polygamy, and a man may divorce his wife simply by saying three times: "I divorce thee." But, Dr. El-Saadwi added, "We are in a difficult transitional phase, and anger must eventually be replaced by an attitude of cooperation and understanding."

India

In early 2001, new census data in India revealed that female fetuses were being aborted at appalling rates. Over the past decade, the population of girls relative to boys tumbled in northern and western India. The census of Punjab, with its large Sikh population, had the lowest proportion of young girls to boys.

Why is the prejudice against girls so prevalent? Some demographers suggest that one reason is that an Indian daughter's responsibility for her parents may end at marriage. In most areas of crowded India, the son usually inherits property, carries on the family line, and is expected to care for aging parents until they die. Then he performs the final service, lighting his parents' funeral pyres to set their souls at peace. A daughter, on the other hand, leaves the natal family after marriage and moves in with her husband's family, sometimes becoming something of a drudge for her in-laws.

The census numbers aroused serious concern and prompted women to promote a campaign against customs such as dowry, property, or money that a girl or woman is expected to bring with her for marriage. Demographers suggest that modernization, better living conditions, and the education of more Indian women physicians may change attitudes.

Indian women have many educational opportunities. Among Indian women who became doctors, the most famous is Anandabai Joshee. When she was born in Poona in 1865, she was named Yamuna. The precocious daughter of a wealthy landed Brahmin, she demanded a tutor to teach her Sanskrit when she was only five years old. When she was nine years old she married a twenty-nine-year-old widower, Gopal Vinyak. She gave up her given name, Yamuna, and became Anandabai.

In 1878 only the most difficult births had the attention of male doctors. Thirteen-year-old Anandabai suffered through a hard delivery and lost her newborn. Grieving, she turned to Christian missionary women who were teaching in India. Her husband approved of her desire to devote her life to alleviating the suffering of Indian women and ignored the outcries of those who opposed the idea. She excelled at her studies and made friends among the nurses and doctors treating patients and encouraging women to study medicine. She impressed the missionaries with her dedication and brilliance. They suggested she apply for admission to an American medical school. She was accepted by the Woman's Medical College of Pennsylvania and became the first unconverted high-cast Hindu woman to leave her home country.

Graduating from the Pennsylvania college in 1886, Anandabai received her degree at a lavish reception in her honor, the first Indian woman with an M.D. anywhere in the world.

Throughout the years of her studies she was plagued by tuberculosis. Many college friends suggested she go to Colorado where the climate and excellent hospital care might improve her health. Though she loved the mountain scenery and the medical staff, she became restless and afraid she might never see her family again. Anandabai made up her mind to risk the long, difficult journey home.

Back in India, the joy of being reunited with her own people temporarily revived her, and she accepted an appointment as physician in charge of the female wards of the Albert Edward Hospital in Kolhapur. By this time, many Indian women doctors were attending patients, both at the hospital and in private practice. Anandabai died at the age of twenty-two, leaving behind a host of remarkable letters.

Japan

Dr. Keiko Okami (1859–1941) was the first Japanese female medical student to study abroad, since it was impossible for a woman in Japan to receive a medical education before World War II. During her lifetime, the terms "woman doctor" and "witch" were synonymous.

Yayoi Yoshioka (1871–1959) founded the Tokyo Women's Medical College, Japan's oldest and longest-surviving training school for women. She became its first president. Insisting that women must have economic independence, she believed medicine would be a path to earn a decent living and to self-respect. Other medical schools admitting women accepted fewer than three or four annually. Some conservative Japanese women continued to oppose medical education for their sisters.

By 1923 the status of Japanese women doctors was not too different from American women practicing in hospitals where they were not staff. By 1950 Aya Kobayashi, born in 1928, passed her national medical examination in Japan. The following year she began her career as a doctor at Yoshida Clinic. There she fulfilled a lifelong dedication to the "eta" people. Her early childhood remembrances were of learning about these special outcasts in Japan who were ostracized. Aya devoted her life to creating compassion and justice for these victims.

China

Most Asian nations are determined to lower their birthrates. Aiming to hold the population to 1.2 billion by the year 2000, China began in 1979 to permit each couple to have a single child. Certain exceptions were made for the one-child family in some rural areas if the firstborn is a daughter.

China's family planning is more effective in cities than in the country, where 85 percent of the population resides. On farms, enforcement appears to be somewhat more lax, and couples have offspring because a farmer needs help with the work. A Chinese farm woman had four daughters in a row. Finally, the family rejoiced with the birth of a son, although the husband was fined a year's salary.

Chinese husbands and wives are required to practice family planning under Article 49 of the 1982 Constitution. An unauthorized pregnancy usually requires an abortion. If a woman gives birth to a second child, in some cases she is sterilized. The sternness of this policy provokes consternation at home and abroad. A new generation is growing up without aunts or uncles.

The population growth rate of China dropped from 2.1 percent to 1.2 percent between 1973 and 2001. Couples committing themselves to one child receive special health care allowances, preferences in admitting the child to good schools, and better access to medical services, jobs, housing, and rural property. Mothers are given longer maternity leaves with pay and without jeopardizing possibilities of promotion.

The *Homiuri shimbun* of Tokyo shocked readers by describing the tragedy of a Chinese woman who lost the younger of her two children, a boy of six, in an accident. The older child was a girl. When the mother became pregnant, a family planning cadre insisted on an abortion. She refused until she was five months pregnant. Then she gave in to harassment and had the abortion. There are records of mothers in rural areas who hide from cadres during their entire pregnancies. Even sadder are mothers who drown baby daughters in the hope the next child will be a boy. In 1994 this attitude changed among the younger generation, particularly among women.

Changes in family size and structure and a longer life span mean that some of China's 1 billion elderly will be without sons or daughters to care for them. Rural China has thousands of old age homes, a situation in a land of filial piety that would have been unthinkable only a few decades ago. In the past, aged peasants without offspring were held in low regard. Today, these elderly folks are nurtured by Chinese women doctors.

In 2001, women with access to ultrasound technology may learn the sex of a child before birth and agree to abort a feminine fetus to please her husband. There is a Chinese tradition of infanticide of girls or denying them nourishment or health care. It is the son who cares for his parents' spirits in the afterlife so "they do not wander for eternity as hungry ghosts." A pregnant woman, seeing beautiful little Chinese girls dressed like dolls, may be encouraged to insist on giving birth to her daughter.

"There's a traditional saying in China," according to Li Shuzhuo, director of the Population Research Center at Xian Jiaotong University in Xian China. "Daughters are like water that splashes out of the family and cannot be gotten back after marriage."

Such insensitivity is not confined to childbirth but has long been evident in the approach to the handicapped who want to become doctors. Highly qualified students were being refused their choice of college or careers for even slight physical handicaps such as a curvature of the spine or poor vision that was actually corrected by glasses.

Lui Wenxiu scored among the top 150 in China's college entrance exams, well over the minimum required at Najing University, a prestigious school. However, she was rejected there and by every university to which she applied simply because she limped. When she applied to a school of traditional medicine, she was informed her scores were too high. Describing Lui's depression in the *New York Times* (May 23, 2001), Elizabeth Rosenthal reported that universities reject disabled applicants because the reputation of the school depends on the rates of the employment of their graduates. Though China's laws against discrimination are strict, the society continues to advertise positions for "tall, young, and thin." Until the close of the twentieth century, education was rarely available for handicapped students. Those disabled students fortunate enough to be educated were often refused admission to college. Chinese universities base acceptance on the results of the national exams. Information about a student's disabilities is included when such results are sent to institutions of higher learning.

Though fortunate to have had excellent schooling, Lui faced insurmountable prejudice in her opportunities for higher education. Eventually, she was encouraged by the Hunan Province Disabled Persons Federation to apply to a junior college dedicated to helping impoverished and disabled students. Though she was accepted and excelled in her courses in finance and economics, she had a nagging concern about the possibility of ever finding a job even after she is fully qualified.

In 1971 Lin Chiao'chih, seventy years old and a leading gynecologist in China, still practiced in the former Peking Union Medicine Center, founded and financed by the Rockefeller Foundation in 1912. She was the first Chinese woman gynecologist to graduate from an English medical school. During her internship, she had been shocked to see American doctors at Peking's Union Medical College experimenting with drugs and bacteria on Chinese patients.

Dr. Lin began her career as a pediatrician but watching babies die broke her heart, so she switched to "bringing them to life." Most mothers gave birth without anesthetics, but in difficult deliveries, anesthesia and other methods were available. Dr. Lin hoped that the need for abortions would be reduced through the distribution of free birth control pills and the teaching of birth control methods in family planning clinics. In the countryside, "barefoot doctors"—barely trained medics—distributed propaganda and the birth control pills that had been developed in China.

In 2001 China was in the grip of widespread discontent, with seriously rising crime and poverty and rampant abduction of women and children.

Ruth V. Hemenway

In the *Medical Woman's Journal* throughout 1945–1947, Ruth Hemenway recorded her observations and experiences as a physician in China. She was born in 1894 and graduated from Tufts Medical School in 1921. Inspired by Dr. Mary Stone lecturing on medical missionary work, Dr. Hemenway made up her mind to go to China. In 1923 she arrived in Fukien Province, and the next year she became superintendent of Mintsing Hospital. She kept a diary of her Chinese experiences from 1923 to 1941.

In 1927, bandits raided the hospital where she was practicing. Though she was terrified, Dr. Hemenway competently treated the villagers who had been attacked.

She assembled a capable staff in 1932 to help develop preventive medicine throughout China. She sugar coated her health programs with skits, songs, lectures, and charts, and taught basic treatments for dysentery, abscesses, tumors, injuries, and newborns. When the Chinese parents of a baby girl offered her their infant for adoption, she promptly accepted. The mother wept. Dr. Hemenway named the infant Huia Sing, which means "Star of China." Cynically, Hmenway recorded, "The mother can have another if she wants to."

She celebrated Christmas 1936 in a newly opened dispensary in the village of South Den near Nanchang. Shortly after, she experienced the terror of war as she and her adopted daughter fled the country.

Margaret H. Polk

Graduating from the Woman's College of Pennsylvania in 1892, Dr. Polk had a private practice in the United States for four years. She had long wanted to work in China and finally fulfilled her desire by going to Soochow to teach in the Women's Medical School. In 1911 she began to feel frustrated by the attitudes of the church toward the women's suffrage movement. Because laity rights were not granted to women, she withdrew from the church and became an independent missionary. In 1913 she set up private practice in Shanghai.

Her niece, Ethel Polk-Peters, graduated from the same Pennsylvania college and joined Polk at the Mary Black Hospital and Woman's Medical College in Soochow. Dr. Polk-Peters organized and inspired Chinese and American women doctors and medical students to work with refugees in Siberia.

5

Women on the March:
Civil War Heroines

There is nothing comparable to the endurance of a woman. In military life, she would tire out an army of men, either in camp or on the march.

Mark Twain, *Autobiography*, 1924

In the nineteenth century, college instruction in medicine had gradually become available to women, but no hospital was willing to provide a woman with an internship or help her pursue a practice. Many of the women who became doctors during this era attended "eclectic" or "homeopathic" schools, which were liberal about accepting women students. Questionable, even cockeyed, theories were taught. Idealistic women often learned as much about temperance, suffrage, and slavery as they did about hygiene or community medicine. Some liberal graduates of these schools became leaders in the abolitionist movement.

Harriot Kezia Hunt

Oliver Wendell Holmes was dean of Harvard University when it became coeducational. Holmes, a brilliant author and physician, had served as professor of anatomy and physiology and had been a Phi Beta Kappa poet at Harvard. In 1850 Harvard Medical College accepted Harriot Kezia Hunt, on her third application. She had practiced medicine without a license for twelve years before applying to Harvard in 1847 and again in 1849. She and her sister Sarah, self-taught in medicine, followed in the footsteps of parents who were "naturalist physicians." Hunt, convinced of the need for qualified women physicians, might have been accepted to Harvard on her second application. But when word got out that she was being considered, hot headed students threatened to transfer to Yale if "female students" were admitted to the medical school.

Very much a Victorian woman, a prisoner of her time and culture, Harriot wrote that she hoped to get from Harvard a "scientific light." Hunt was no activist, but when

Harvard dismissed her application as "inexpedient," she joined a women's rights movement. Informed that Elizabeth Blackwell had been accepted to a medical college, Hunt resubmitted a third application with a reminder that women were determined to practice medicine. Shouldn't they be encouraged to get good training? She added that the refusal "in the city of my birth, education, and life, seemed unjust to me." Perhaps Holmes's support for her application was influenced by a photograph that showed her as a matronly overweight woman, unlikely to arouse sexual longing in any fellow student. She was accepted, along with three black applicants. These four students were discriminated against from the word "go." They were allowed to attend lectures, but they should not expect to earn a degree.

Harvard students were not the liberals then that they became a century later. The men opposed the very idea that Hunt would be permitted in the medical lecture room "where her presence is calculated to destroy our respect for the modesty and delicacy of her sex." As for the "socially repulsive blacks," the men felt justified in staging a riot to protect "the dignity of the college."

Harriot Hunt was forced to withdraw. To its shame, Harvard passed a resolution prohibiting the admission of women, a policy enforced until 1946.

Irene S. Toland

After the outbreak of the brief Spanish-American War that arose out of Spain's policies in Cuba, Dr. Irene Toland went to nurse the wounded of Teddy Roosevelt's Rough Riders. She was there during Roosevelt's famous charge up San Juan Hill. During the battle, she was wounded. Though bleeding, she continued tending the soldiers who required medical care. Born in 1857 into a prominent southern family, Irene grew up on her father's plantation, destined for a protected comfortable existence, "a flower of the weaker sex." However, as a young woman, Irene Toland felt a call to a life of service as a missionary. Both she and her brother, John, named for his father, studied to be physicians.

On a trip to Mexico, she recognized the crying need for a clinic and primary school. With gutsy determination, and almost single-handedly, she launched both projects. When her sister, Rebecca, offered to operate the school and clinic, Toland agreed. She had already determined she would try to repeat her success in Cuba. She arrived just about the time war broke out. She died of her injuries and is buried in the Old Masonic Cemetery in Washington County, Texas. The message on her tombstone reads, "She died a martyr to the duty to which she believed she was divinely called."

Civil War Heroines

Clara Barton

During the Civil War, Clara Barton became known as the "American Florence Nightingale" and "the Angel of the Battlefield." A born nurse and a dynamic organizer, Barton won the support of Union generals and brought supplies to the front and compassion to troops on both sides of the war. Her courage to overcome almost insurmountable odds led to the founding of the American Red Cross—to serve, not only in wartime, but in times of natural disasters as well.

Born Christmas Day, 1821, in North Oxford, Massachusetts, Clara, the fifth child of a thirty-eight-year old mother, was welcomed into a family who supported the abolitionist movement. Her mother held that "women deserve perfectly equal rights—human rights."

When Clara's brother, David, was dangerously ill, she nursed him back to health. Later, he taught her to ride horseback. During the Civil War years later, when she had to ride a strange horse, she was "flying for life. I blessed the early gallops."

Clara started teaching in a one-room school at seventeen. She had forty students. Barton's school received the highest standing for discipline in North Oxford. The following year, she was offered a salary less than that the school board paid men. She responded, "If paid at all, I shall never do a man's work for less than a man's pay." She was paid what she demanded. Years later, at her insistence, a new free public school was opened in Bordentown, New Jersey, where she taught 200 students and had them read Harriet Beecher Stowe's *Uncle Tom's Cabin.*

In 1854 she moved to Washington and became the only woman employed in the Patent Office. Barton heard Lincoln's Inaugural Address on the Capitol steps and remembered it the rest of her life.

When Fort Sumter fell to Southern troops in April 1861, neither barracks nor hospitals had been prepared. Barton learned that the wounded were being housed in the Senate Chamber of the Capitol. The soldiers had lost all their baggage. Though it was Sunday, she convinced merchants to open their shops and allow her to buy baskets of food, and she hired porters to carry everything to the Capitol. The next day she advertised in the newspaper, asking readers to send supplies. The response was so overwhelming, she had to rent three warehouses. She needed a pass to get these supplies to the front, and several frustrating months passed before she could obtain one.

The normal order of a military train was ammunition first, then food and clothing, and last, hospital supplies. Clara manipulated her drivers to get her medical supplies to arrive ahead of the ammunition. The only woman at the Battle of Antietam, she drove the men to unload her crates of lanterns, clean linen, bandages, and medicine. In a barn converted to a hospital, Barton took her place next to the doctors. She administered chloroform and dressed wounds. "You saved my life," she heard repeatedly.

At Fredericksburg in 1862, she faced the greatest challenge of her life. Arriving by boat in a drenching downpour, she was hurried to the Old National Hotel where hundreds of wounded and dying lay on wet bloody floors. For four days and nights, hardly stopping to eat, she stood beside a surgeon who amputated hands, arms, and legs. While Clara was a guest at a candlelit dinner in a Fredericksburg home, she received permission to have the wounded moved into the house. Logs soon blazed in the fireplaces, and decent food was prepared for the injured men.

In 1863 Clara's favorite brother, David, was ordered to Hilton Head, South Carolina. Clara requested permission from the War Department to join him. In a beautiful house, they ate with officers glittering with gold braid. Barton enjoyed fine food and elegant service, and the company of a genteel colonel, John J. Elwell, who had a broken leg. Barton, in her battlefield experiences, had despised the privileges of officers and their arrogant disregard for human life. Overcoming her resentment, she enjoyed the humor and attention of the colonel. They rode horseback in the early mornings. The colonel called her "Birdie" and wrote her that he "loved her all the law allowed." While the sounds of guns of the Union Army pounding Fort Sumter kept the horror of war alive, her response to Elwell's poetic courtship made her happy; however, she knew he was married. When Clara left Hilton Head, Elwell made sure she had a saddle horse and an ambulance with a "good bed and what she needed to keep house."

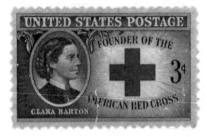

One of a set of stamps honoring Clara Barton, issued in 1948.

The South surrendered in 1865, but the agony of the war was not over for the Bartons. They had lost touch with Stephen Barton for years. Finally, Clara learned that he was a prisoner and dangerously sick. Clara's reputation for all she had done for the Union helped find him. She nursed him, but he died soon after.

She grieved for him, but at least she knew what had happened to him. After returning to Washington, she received thousands of letters from families without a clue to what had happened to a husband, son, or brother. She organized a Washington bureau to search for missing military men. A letter from Dorence Atwater, a New Englander, said he was captured shortly after joining the army. He had endured twenty-two months in Andersonville Prison. Because he had fine handwriting, he had been assigned to keep records of name, rank, and cause of death of every prisoner; he had recorded 700 a week. He suspected the Confederacy would try to hide evidence of brutal treatment of prisoners, so he kept both an official register for the South and one for himself. His own copy, made at night, he hid in the lining of his jacket. Without a name, each grave had been marked only by a small numbered stick. After the war, he smuggled north the number that marked a soldier's place in the long rows of trench graves. Barton acquired Atwater's lists, and using them with her massive correspondence, located more than 22,000 missing soldiers in four years. With these graves marked, Barton asked that the former prison grounds be converted to a national cemetery at Andersonville. In 1865, the task completed, she raised the flag at a dedication.

Perhaps the first woman ever to testify before Congress, she so impressed the all-male body with her achievements in this sad project at her own expense that they appropriated $15,000 to continue her work.

On a lecture tour in the winter of 1868, Clara collapsed on the stage. Her doctors recommended a trip to Europe. In Geneva, she read a book, *Un Souvenir de Solerino* (A Memory of Solferino), by Henri Dunant, a Swiss humanitarian. He had been in northern Italy in 1859 when French and Italian soldiers clashed with Austrians in the battle of Solferino. Dunant, shocked by the wounds or deaths of some 40,000 combatants, bought medical supplies and organized hospitalization. He began an intensive campaign for societies of volunteers to rescue the war wounded without regard to nationality.

Barton learned about the Treaty of Geneva, signed by sixteen nations in 1864, stipulating that hospitals flying a Red Cross flag would not be fired on or captured. Surgeons, nurses, and chaplains would be regarded as neutrals and expected to help victims on either side of a war. Badly wounded soldiers would not be imprisoned but returned instead to their own army. Barton successfully appealed for American approval of the treaty.

When the daughter of King Wilhelm of Prussia requested aid in distributing relief from Red Cross warehouses for the garrisoned city of Strasbourg, Barton rushed to help. On the way to Strasbourg, she removed a red ribbon she wore at her throat and made a cross of it to sew on her sleeve. She became the first American ever to wear the insignia of the International Red Cross.

In the burned ruins of devastated Strasbourg in September 1870, some 6,000 homeless, starving people crawled out of cellars. With her own funds, Clara appealed to Americans to send clothing or fabric and patterns. She set up workrooms where women made or altered the clothes. On Christmas Eve 1871, Barton, summoned to her door, was greeted by the entire population of Strasbourg to celebrate her fiftieth birthday with a tree decorated with candles glittering like stars.

In 1873 she returned to the United States to promote the idea of an American Red Cross to be included in the Treaty of Geneva. She campaigned for the American Red Cross also to include relief for victims of national disasters. When Barton approached President James A. Garfield, a Civil War veteran, and asked him to become the first president of the Association of the American Red Cross, he urged Clara to take the post herself. In 1881 she was elected president and held that position until 1904. In 1884 in Geneva, she represented the United States at the International Red Cross conference and from then on in Karlsruhe, Rome, Vienna, and St. Petersburg.

Her European humanitarian work brought extraordinary awards, among them the Jewel of the Red Cross of Serbia, the Gold Cross of Remembrance from the Grand Duke of Baden, and the Iron Cross of Merit from Kaiser Wilhelm. In old age, she wore all her medals on her apron when she did her gardening. Barton died at home in Glen Echo, Maryland, in 1912 at the age of ninety.

Esther Hill Hawks

When Esther Hill Hawks tried to volunteer to serve in the Union Army, she was rejected as a doctor but agreed to be a nurse. In South Carolina, her physician husband, taking care of the wounded, was promoted to head of a hospital for black soldiers, most of whom had been freed by Union forces. Overwhelmed by the number of wounded, he summoned his wife. Esther joined her husband to care for the First South Carolina Volunteers, the first official black regiment in the Union Army. In 1863, 150 wounded were brought in after a fierce battle at Fort Wagner. Esther was shocked at the sight of these black soldiers so "mangled and ghastly." She found many college graduates in the regiment "intelligent, courteous, cheerful and kind . . . I pity the humanity which . . . retains the unworthy prejudice against color!" she wrote.

Throughout the Civil War, trained nurses worked side by side with untrained women who came to tent hospitals that were steaming hot in summer and freezing cold in winter. Few tents had wood floors. Often a woman who was neither nurse nor doctor would come to a hospital to care for her own son or husband. Frequently, out of the goodness of her heart, she tended other wounded as well.

The women who helped nurse the sick and wounded were called "laundresses." They washed and boiled linens and uniforms, cooked, and mended. Most importantly, they were competent nurses working without salary until the Army Nursing Corps was established and nurses began to receive $12 a month, army rations, and free travel.

Mary Edwards Walker

A little-known Civil War army doctor, Mary Edwards Walker graduated at twenty-two, from Syracuse Medical College in 1855, the only woman in her class. Walker's certificate from the short-lived college did not have the respect eventually given Elizabeth Blackwell's degree from Geneva Medical College. However, Walker was accepted by the Union Army in 1861—if she would volunteer her services. Women as nurses or doctors were not commissioned until three years later, when Dr. Walker became acting assistant surgeon and a first lieutenant. She claimed to be the first woman to serve on the surgical staff of any modern army in wartime.

Born in 1832, Mary was educated by her parents. Her father, Alvah Walker, was a doctor and taught Mary how to treat farm animals as well as his patients. Proof exists in War Department documents that Dr. Walker was captured by the Confederates near Chattanooga. She spent four months under cruel conditions in terrible prisons. Walker was constantly harassed by her male colleagues. Nevertheless, she was able to have a lasting effect on the Confederate prison by insisting that wheat bread and fresh vegetables be substituted for salt pork and corn bread. Eventually she and twenty-four other Union doctors were traded for seventeen Confederate surgeons.

Recuperating from her ordeal, she remained with the Union Army. She organized an association to help women find relatives and friends among soldiers in Washington, D.C. For pregnant women, Walker always lent a helping hand and a sympathetic ear.

When Walker saw that much mail was being dumped because it could neither be delivered nor returned, she carried on a campaign to have all envelopes carry a return address and all registered mail have a return receipt. The suggestion at the time was seen as enormously innovative.

For her untiring service "on the field of duty," President Abraham Lincoln recommended the Medal of Honor. She did not receive it until 1865 from President Andrew Johnson. Despite the citation from Lincoln, people called Dr. Walker crazy. She had cut off her hair to sell for a soldier's wife who was destitute and homeless in Washington, a city overrun by crippled and dying soldiers. Dr. Walker adopted pants during her years in uniform. She wore pants to her wedding ceremony with Albert Miller and refused to take her husband's name. She insisted that any vow to obey her husband be omitted from the ceremony. The marriage didn't last long.

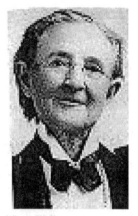

Not only did she have a medical degree, but Mary Walker also had studied law, and she used her legal knowledge to counsel the poverty-stricken veterans and their dependents to get pensions. She opened a sanitarium and survived with one foot on a soapbox, giving public lectures on the prevention of tuberculosis and the dangers of smoking and liquor. She deplored capital punishment and campaigned for women's suffrage and the right of women to dress as they pleased. Eventually, the public regarded her as a freak lecturing at dime museums for her living.

In a spiteful letter to the *New York Medical Journal* in 1867, Captain Robert Bartholow accused Dr. Walker of being a spy and informer. The captain claimed "she had no more medical knowledge than any ordinary housewife." That Mary Walker was ever a spy is highly unlikely. As to the accusation that she had no more

Mary Walker was recommended for the Medal of Honor by President Abraham Lincoln. *(Photo courtesy of Library of Congress.)*

knowledge of medicine than most housewives, neither did most male doctors of the time. Conservatives criticized Dr. Walker's militancy and lifestyle, but she continued to teach, write books, and fight for women's rights. Two years before her death in 1917, the award of the Medal of Honor was reversed. That year, guidelines for receiving the award were revised so that only a man who had carried a weapon and engaged in combat could receive the Medal of Honor. Walker adamantly refused to return her medal, even though she was stripped of the right to have it.

Attitudes toward feminism had changed by 1977. The issue of her Medal of Honor that had been revoked sixty years earlier again came up in Congress. An army review board recommended restoring the medal. A United States postage stamp was issued in her honor. Dr. Walker died at eighty-seven, penniless and ostracized by her family. Congress and history restored her reputation.

Mother Bickerdyke and Mary Safford

On a cold wet November day in 1861, Mary Ann Bickerdyke and Mary Safford waited on a slippery dock for a journalist, Anna Ella Carroll, whose reports made a substantial contribution to the record of the role of women in the Civil War. Bickerdyke and Stafford had appointed themselves as an informal reception committee for the writer, who was well-known for her political articles in an age when women rarely spoke or wrote about world problems. Women, if they wrote about anything, were expected to discuss cooking, housekeeping, and child rearing or produce poetry and romantic fiction.

Bickerdyke drew her cloak close against the cold wind. She was eager to meet this "Carroll woman" because she knew President Abraham Lincoln had asked Carroll to go down the Mississippi River into the heart of enemy territory and report her impressions to him.

In a camp kitchen, the three women sat with tea and talked long into the night. Carroll wanted to know all about Bickerdyke. "You're famous," Miss Carroll said.

The reporter learned that Mary Ann was born on a farm in Knox County, Ohio, in 1817. Her mother died when she was only seventeen months old. For a few years, Mary Ann lived with her grandparents in Richland County, Ohio. Then she moved from one relative to another. Before she was a teenager, she was already a servant in the home of strangers. She married a forty-one-year-old widower with several children. Robert Bickerdyke, a native of England, painted signs and houses for a living. He loved music and dreamed of a musical career. Mary Ann proved to be a good mother to his children, and she gave birth to two sons. The third baby, a daughter, Martha, died when she was only two. The loss of this little girl made Mary Ann wonder if she could have saved her child if she had known more about medicine. She longed to be a doctor, even though she knew women were not accepted to medical school.

In 1859 she was left a widow, the sole support of her children and stepchildren. She began to study botanic medicine, a therapy using drugs made of vegetable juices, bark, roots, and herbs. When Carroll asked Bickerdyke where she had learned practical nursing, Bickerdyke replied that she was self-taught.

"And what brought you here?"

In 1861 Mary Ann Bickerdyke had heard the Rev. Edward Beecher in the Galesburg Congregational Church describe the terrible neglect of young Illinois soldiers suffering from dysentery and typhoid at a camp in Cairo, Illinois. The church congregation raised a relief fund. But Bickerdyke wanted to give more than money. She wanted to give herself. Arriving at her first camp in Cairo, Bickerdyke could smell the stench a mile away. In many camps, the men did not dig latrines but used the woods. The water supply was dangerously filthy. Bickerdyke saw mountains of garbage, dead dogs, and a pile of amputated arms and legs. Working like a demon, she stripped the filthy, bloody battle clothes from the wounded, bathed them, and boiled their towels and clothes. She was called "a cyclone in calico."

She became superintendent of the hospital in Cairo, where everyone knew her affectionately as "Mother Bickerdyke."

The reporter, turning to Mary Jane Safford, asked, "Where are you from?"

"I was born in Hyde Park, Vermont, but I grew up in Crete, Illinois. I went to school there and in Vermont and Montreal. I live with my older brother. I heard of an epidemic killing volunteer troops. I came to the camp to take care of the sick men."

When young Mary Safford, wealthy and well educated, arrived at the Belmont battlefield, in the little village south of Cairo, General Grant had blundered and barely won the day. Thousands of slaughtered men lay everywhere. Safford went from one fallen soldier to the next, feeling for a pulse. She spoke encouragingly to each one who had a heartbeat and promised to get him to a hospital. When a bullet whizzed past her, she dropped flat on her face. Another bullet passed just above her head. She reached for a small branch of a tree, a twig, really, and tied her handkerchief to it. Waving her white flag of truce, she rose and continued to kneel by the wounded, promising to get help to them.

The rancid odor of frying grease made the air putrid. Men were issued salt pork, coffee, beans, and tobacco. Fresh fruits and vegetables were rarely seen in camp. The soldiers drank water wherever they found it. Because the water could be contaminated, Safford encouraged them to drink hot tea or coffee; at least the water would be boiled.

She did not have the energy to keep up with the whirlwind pace of Bickerdyke, but the two were close friends. Safford had taught school until 1861, when Cairo was occupied by Grant's soldiers in the hastily erected camps. Safford never objected to Bickerdyke's strong language and earthy manners because Safford respected the older woman's dedication.

When the reporter asked, "Do the officers cooperate with you?" Bickerdyke went into a tirade, her angry target the corrupt medical officers. She also condemned lay orderlies. She wanted an orderly sent back to battle if he sat around smoking, playing cards, or drinking. As soon as a soldier could stand on his own feet, she expected him to help care for the more seriously wounded who lay in cots around him.

One day, an indignant doctor asked Mother Bickerdyke: "Who gave you the authority to use those supplies?" She answered, "My authority comes from God. Do you have anyone ranking higher than that?"

Carroll, hearing this oft-repeated story, smiled because she knew about the night Colonel John A. Logan, a wounded congressman from Illinois, looked out of the flap of his tent and spotted a figure moving close to the ground across the dark forbidding battlefield. "Who is that?" he wondered. He knew that robbers stripped the dead and wounded. The colonel sent his orderly to stop whoever or whatever was carrying on out there. The soldier returned with Mother Bickerdyke. In her brash country manner, she exploded, "Some soldiers in the frozen mud may be still alive. Do you expect me to sleep?"

She had little faith in stretcher-bearers, who might not look for the wounded under a shrub or thicket or in a ravine. Even the bearers were exhausted. On such a freezing night, a man might still be breathing and be so cold he could be passed up as a corpse. Mother Bickerdyke, wrapped in a heavy shawl and carrying her lantern, went out to look for herself. From that time on, Colonel Logan was Bickerdyke's friend and ally.

The story of Mother Bickerdyke made headlines in all the newspapers that carried Anna Ella Carroll's byline. Bickerdyke learned that Carroll was a Southerner sympathetic to the Union and to Lincoln's desire to free the slaves. Her family had already freed all their slaves, at great financial sacrifice.

Bickerdyke told the reporter that it was more dangerous to be brought to a military hospital than to be taken home in a jouncing horse-drawn carriage. Stretcher-bearers brought a steady stream of wounded men. Hospital supplies ran out. Safford said, "Sometimes we run out of morphine. Our wounded who require surgery get some kind of anesthesia, usually ether."

Carroll said, "In the South, our medical tradition came from the French. Chloroform is more popular. Many field surgeons on both sides in the war use chloroform because it acts quickly."

Safford believed chloroform was more dangerous than ether. Soldiers died from too much of it. When the supply of chloroform was exhausted, she and Bickerdyke encouraged the patient to drink a glass of whiskey.

Bickerdyke became one of the most famous Civil War heroines, a friend of General Ulysses Grant and of General William T. Sherman. Sherman respected Bickerdyke and would not hear a word of criticism of her, though he scolded her. Mother Bickerdyke, now matron of the military hospital in Memphis, was heartsick over the shortages of eggs, meat, milk, butter, and fresh fruits and vegetables. In 1862 and again in 1864, her speaking tour of cities in the Midwest and the North resulted in receptive audiences contributing everything she needed, including bushels of potatoes, onions, live chickens, ducks, even cows and pigs delivered to the trains. Farmers worried that their livestock would not safely get to the soldiers, because after all, a live animal requires food, water, care, and a clean pen. However, Bickerdyke got all the animals transported—healthy, noisy, and troublesome—to Memphis.

Later, near Vicksburg, Bickerdyke joined Grant's army and may have saved the lives of hundreds of wounded men. She did not sleep or rest until every wounded soldier had been cleaned, bandaged, and given a hot meal and a hot drink.

Sherman intended to capture Atlanta where four important railroads had a junction. The loss of the city, with its foundries, arsenals, and machine shops, could be the death knell of the Confederacy. Sherman captured the city, but the Confederate Army escaped.

In 1863 Sherman saw how exhausted Bickerdyke had become, and he sent her home. She rejoined the army at the Battle of Missionary Ridge and assembled barrels of food and bandages at Nashville for the spring campaign of 1864. She learned that Sherman had commanded that nothing but military articles could travel on the railroad from Nashville. Bickerdyke decided that if a mule-drawn train of ambulances was not to carry barrels, she would empty supplies into bags and get them on the ambulances. In defiance of Sherman's order against noncombatant passengers on the railroad, she bullied her way onto the next train to Chattanooga. She shoved aside aides trying to stop her and stormed in to see Sherman. "May I come in, General?"

"I should think you had got in," growled Sherman.

"General, I can't stand this last order of yours. You'll have to change it as sure as you live. . . . After a man is unable to carry a gun and drops out of the line, you don't trouble yourself about him but turn him over to the hospitals. . . . We must have supplies." Sherman said he was busy. Bickerdyke replied: "Fix things as it ought to be fixed. Have some sense about it!" Sherman laughed, and they talked reasonably to each other. Bickerdyke said, "Well, I can't stand fooling here all day. . . . Write an order for two cars a day." General Sherman did so at once.

Bickerdyke followed the army from Chattanooga with a traveling laundry. She and her aides changed bandages, cleaned wounds, and bathed the men. When hot water was scarce, she did not empty the tub after bathing a wounded major general but followed up with bathing fifteen privates in the same water! Army surgeons accused her of getting in the way and crowding hospitals with relief supplies not on the military list. Sherman's response to the surgeons' complaints was "She outranks me. I can't do a thing in the world."

In 1864, Bickerdyke, raising funds at charity affairs, read in the newspaper that Sherman's army had reached Savannah. She hurried through the last speech and did not wait for questions but rushed to board a coastal steamer with a load of supplies. The ship docked in Wilmington, North Carolina, and Bickerdyke disembarked to comfort the last remnants of a small band of Union soldiers who had been incarcerated in the terrible Andersonville prisoner-of-war compound. Her heart went out to these emaciated men who looked like walking dead. They were amused and astounded at the blustering biddy who had an encouraging word for every soldier. She challenged them to get well, go home, and live a normal life. Later, Mother Bickerdyke joined the main battalion of the army at Beaufort, North Carolina, where she was nursing the wounded when peace was declared in 1865.

Bickerdyke, honored in the great victory parade in Washington, rode among Sherman's triumphant forces. Those who saw her in the parade and remembered her fund-raising speeches cheered her, shouted her name, and waved American flags.

Bickerdyke moved west and ran a boardinghouse along the new Kansas Pacific Railroad. Veterans moved to the area to settle on Kansas farmland. Sometime around 1869, Bickerdyke met Sherman on a street in the capital and told him she was strapped for money to pay for an extension on her mortgage. He took her case to the railroad magnates and obtained an extension, but in the end, she lost the house. She moved to New York and worked for Protestant charities until 1874, then moved back to Kansas to be near her two sons. She became active in helping victims of a locust plague. Like Walt Whitman, who had also nursed the wounded, Mother Bickerdyke saw the necessity for soldiers to receive pensions. She made repeated trips to Washington to promote the idea, and was grateful when Congress granted her a pension of $25 a month in 1886. She died in 1901.

With the war over, Mary Safford considered going to medical school. Mary had the formal education to be accepted, but she was exhausted from her years of nursing the wounded. She richly enjoyed a grand tour of Europe and came home determined to be a physician. In 1869 she graduated from New York Medical College for Women, founded by Dr. Elizabeth Blackwell. She could afford advanced training in Europe, and for three years she studied at the General Hospital of Vienna and at a number of German medical centers. At the University of Breslau, Safford was the first woman to perform an ovariotomy. In 1872 she opened private practice in Chicago. When she met a Boston man who respected and loved her, she accepted his proposal. Contented and fulfilled, she moved her practice to his city and became a professor of women's diseases at the Boston University of Medicine. She was a staff physician as well at the Massachusetts Homeopathic Hospital. Promotion of public education in health and hygiene led to her election in 1875 to the Boston School Committee. She continued practicing medicine until 1886 when she moved to Florida. She died in 1891.

6

Pioneers, O Pioneers!:
Then and Now

> *O you young and elder daughters!*
> *O you mothers and you wives!*
> *Never must you be divided,*
> *in our ranks you move united,*
> *Pioneers, O, Pioneers!*
>
> Walt Whitman, *Leaves of Grass*

Two women in the nineteenth century evoked great changes in the role of women in medicine. Florence Nightingale, born in Florence, Italy, in 1820, developed the concept of the completely trained nurse. Elizabeth Blackwell, born in Bristol, England, in 1821, is famous as America's first woman physician, but it is not so well-known that she was also the first accredited woman doctor of Great Britain. A decade after she had received her diploma from Geneva College in New York, Elizabeth Blackwell was enrolled as a recognized physician in the Medical Register of the United Kingdom. Indeed, she was the first woman ever to achieve this honor. Soon after, Dr. Blackwell met with Nightingale and discussed her recently published *Notes on Hospitals*, the book that revolutionized the theory of hospital construction and management. Blackwell was interested in a proposed Nightingale Training School for Nurses at St. Thomas's Hospital that would open in 1860.

Florence Nightingale

Florence was named for the city of her birth and was educated in mathematics and the classics at home under the guidance of her father. Discontented with the social life of her upper-class family, she began studying hospitals in 1844. On a trip that included Egypt, she met two nursing nuns of St. Vincent de Paul in

Alexandria who encouraged her interest in improving schools and hospitals. A year later she studied at the institute for Protestant deaconesses in Kaiserswerth, Germany, and followed up with specialized nursing in Paris. In 1853, appointed superintendent of the Hospital for Invalid Gentlewomen in London, she was responsible for improving the hospital.

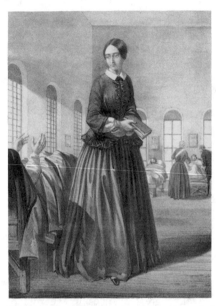

The Nightingale's Song to the Sick and Wounded (Photo courtesy of the Philadelphia Museum of Art, The William H. Helfand Collection.)

In 1854, England, France, and Turkey were at war with Russia. Troops had landed in the Crimea without medical supplies. England learned that the barracks hospital in Scutari was execrable. The French had sent Sisters of Charity, but the British had not provided care for the sick or wounded. Nightingale wrote her friend, Sidney Herbert, secretary of war, volunteering to organize nurses for army hospitals. He had also written to her asking that she go to the Crimea; their letters crossed in the mail. He promised complete cooperation of the medical staff there. Nightingale quickly recruited ten Catholic nuns, fourteen Anglican sisters, and fourteen regular hospital nurses, and they were on their way to Scutari. A few days before their arrival, transports of wounded from the Battle of Balaclava had been brought to the hospital. The men lay untended on reeking straw mattresses crawling with vermin. Only weeks later, 1,800 more men were wounded in the bloody Battle of Inkerman. Nightingale had to contend with official hostility against women in military hospitals while on her feet twenty hours at a time caring for the wounded or assisting in the operating room. Nightingale tended four miles of beds all day. Into the dawn she wrote reports for Sidney Herbert.

Her constant wrestling with red tape and military authorities proved to be an overwhelming challenge. The commissariat regarded her as a dangerous innovator and thwarted her every effort.

She wrote Herbert that military hospitals had to be reorganized and the need to keep medical statistics was imperative. She proposed that an army medical school be established immediately in Turkey. Many young surgeons at that time came into service with no training in military medicine or camp hygiene. This situation had to change.

In England her name became a revered household word. Through Longfellow's poem "Filomena," she became known everywhere as "The Lady with the Lamp."

At the end of the Crimean War, England wanted to forget the agony of it quickly. Florence Nightingale would never forget the soldiers in "an old pair of regimental trousers, fed on raw salt meat . . . nine thousand lying, from causes which might have been prevented, in their forgotten graves!"

The queen and prince consort, summering at Balmoral Castle, invited Miss Nightingale to visit and thanked her personally for her services in the Crimean War. The famous nurse asked for a formal investigation of unhealthy conditions in the British army. Prince Albert wrote in his diary that Nightingale detailed all the defects of the system and the needed reforms, and he promised action.

The queen remarked, "Such a head! I wish we had her at the War Office!"

True to the prince's assurance, a Royal Commission was established to study the barracks in which the death rate among soldiers was at least twice and in some places five times as great as that of the nonmilitary populations living in the same areas.

Florence Nightingale would not rest until the War Office remodeled military hospitals and barracks, improved the diet, and made the drinking water safe. In the Army Medical School, the training of doctors was transformed.

Until 1859, when Nightingale campaigned to make civilian hospitals keep uniform statistics about their patients, records had been sketchy and inadequate. She drew up model statistical forms and persuaded Sir James Page of St. Bartholomew's Hospital to try them for a year. By the end of the year, they proved so valuable that they were adopted not only by St. Bartholomew's but also by most London hospitals and eventually throughout the civilized world.

The concept of the completely trained nurse developed by Nightingale became a reality at the St. Thomas Hospital when probationers began studies in the Nightingale School of Nursing in 1860. Nightingale's crusade to improve hospitals and professional nursing was based on her principle that "the very first requirement in a hospital must be that it should do the sick no harm." Nightingale became a world authority on hospital construction and management. In 1876 she sent complete plans for a projected hospital to Johns Hopkins University in Baltimore, and not a single suggestion she made was rejected. She was eighty-seven in 1907 when she was awarded the British Order of Merit, the first woman ever to receive that honor. Five years after her death in 1910, the Crimean Monument was erected in Waterloo Place, London, in her honor.

Elizabeth Blackwell

In 1767 the University of Pennsylvania launched the first American medical school. No one dreamed of admitting a woman. Historian John B. Blake noted that the only careers that an educated woman might aspire to were writing (for the talented few) and teaching. School boards discovered that women might be hired at half the salary they paid men, and a rapid rise in the number of women teachers began in 1820. A generation of ambitious women who later became famous started their professional lives as teachers. Among them was Elizabeth

Blackwell. In her autobiography, *Pioneer Work in Opening the Medical Profession to Women*, she documented her lifelong fight against prejudice.

Her British father, a sugar refiner who had been active in the antislavery struggle in England, expected the family to give up sugar because it was a "slave product." British governesses and masters had tutored the nine children and encouraged a passion for reading. Of the children, the two older girls, Elizabeth and Emily, were in their teens when the family migrated to New York. Elizabeth enrolled in a fine school and soon became involved in the antislavery struggle. She was seventeen when the Blackwell family moved to Cincinnati and joined the Unitarian Church, which was active in the freedom movement. The girls appreciated Harriet Beecher Stowe's books, especially *Uncle Tom's Cabin*. Within a few months after the move west, tragedy struck the family. The summer heat was too much for Mr. Blackwell's English constitution, and he died of fever, leaving a widow and nine children in poverty. The three older daughters opened a day school for girls and supported the family. Elizabeth, bored with teaching, considered studying to be a midwife because obstetrics was still a woman's profession.

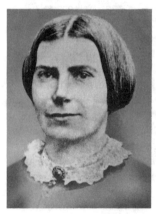

In 1849 Elizabeth Blackwell graduated from Geneva College of Medicine. *(Photo courtesy of New York Infirmary.)*

Blackwell admits she was "ashamed of any form of illness, and considered sickness contemptible." As a girl, she tried to harden her body by sleeping on the floor. When a teacher tried to enliven a lesson by passing around a bull's eye, Elizabeth almost vomited. So what led this woman to study medicine? Repeatedly she was told she had an unrealistic goal. She observed, "The idea of winning a doctor's degree gradually assumed the aspect of a great moral struggle." She was angry that the term "woman physician" came to mean an abortionist and a crude one at that. Hired as a governess for the children of a North Carolina doctor, she studied his books in her spare time, squirreling away money until 1847 when she applied for acceptance to medical schools. Because Philadelphia was then considered the seat of medical learning, she moved there and boarded with Dr. William Elder's family. Doctors who interviewed her offered only discouragement. "You can't expect us to furnish you with a stick to break our head with," a dean told her. Another professor suggested a partnership with Elizabeth on the condition that she share profits over $5,000 on her first year's practice. A dean suggested she might be accepted to medical school if she disguised herself as a man. The first English woman doctor, James (Miranda) Berry, was discovered to be a woman only after she died in 1865. She had practiced all her life in the guise of a man and had been so highly respected that she became inspector general of hospitals for the British army.

Blackwell, while applying to colleges, studied anatomy in a private school. One of her first lessons involved the human wrist. "The beauty of the tendons and the exquisite arrangement of this part of the body" so appealed to her that she never again felt the repulsion she had known in handling the bull's eye. In 1847, when she was accepted by Geneva College of Medicine in New York, she was overjoyed. One of Blackwell's medical classmates recalled the amazement in the lecture hall when a woman student walked in. "Her entrance into a bedlam of confusion acted like magic. For the first time, a lecture was given without the slightest interruption, and every word could be heard as distinctly as if there had been a single person in the room." The sudden transformation of this class from a band of lawless desperadoes to gentlemen by the mere presence of a lady proved to be permanent in its effect.

Elizabeth Blackwell, urged to refrain from attending lectures on the reproductive system, replied in writing to the professor. She said that anatomy, a serious study, "reflected glory on the Creator." The professor reconsidered. When she entered the hall, her fellow students gave her a standing ovation. A classmate remembered that thereafter, the lectures on anatomy were delivered in much better taste, for it was well-known that this professor enjoyed off-color jokes and wisecracks.

In the two years she studied in Geneva, her enthusiasm for medicine grew. It was an era when any male with an elementary education could take lecture courses for a winter or two, pass an examination, and achieve the right to practice medicine. For some doctors, their entire education lasted less than a year. As late as 1900, medical schools admitted students who were rejected by liberal arts colleges.

Fellow medical students respected Blackwell, and four of them volunteered to do extra dissection with her at night under the supervision of an anatomy professor. Often the group worked until after midnight, when Elizabeth returned to her little room to make notes. Most of the students accepted Elizabeth without reservation, but the townspeople seemed to resent her. Some women crossed the street when they saw her coming. Some spread rumors that Elizabeth was crazy. Other residents of her boardinghouse gave her the silent treatment at meals. At the end of the first term, Elizabeth Blackwell returned to Philadelphia and was able to get permission to work at a grim hospital for the poor, Blockley Almshouse. There, older doctors were helpful to the pale blond beauty, but young residents openly resented her. Whenever Elizabeth walked into a ward, the young men walked out, carrying away all the charts that provided diagnosis and treatment of ward patients. Elizabeth was left on her own to study the cases. But the young students were actually doing her a favor.

She needed to write a graduation thesis. The disastrous potato famine of 1848 gave her a subject. Boatloads of malnourished Irish immigrants arriving in America became patients at Blockley Almshouse. Elizabeth wrote her thesis on typhus. Her research on these victims was hailed as a major contribution to medicine, yet a lively discussion continued on whether or not Geneva College could actually confer the degree of doctor of medicine on a female.

On the morning of January 23, 1849, Elizabeth Blackwell dressed for commencement. Some of her warmest supporters on the faculty were in their glory. Many Geneva women came to see her receive a medical diploma. With pounding heart, Blackwell, elegant in a black silk brocade gown, green gloves, and black silk stockings, watched her fellow graduates, four at a time, ascend the steps to the platform and ceremoniously receive diplomas. A brass band in Indian costumes provided the graduation music. Left to the very last, Elizabeth Blackwell was called up alone. The president removed his hat and handed her the diploma.

Feminine, modest, and graceful, she decided to speak, and did so with dignity. "It shall be the effort of my life to shed honor on this diploma," she said. The audience applauded in approval. Nodding gravely, the faculty joined the applause. The next announcement was that Blackwell had graduated at the head of her class.

Dr. Blackwell, determined to learn more about medicine, decided to return to England to work at Lying-in Hospital. She was a curiosity in England. A British humor magazine, *Punch*, published a long poem in her honor. One of its verses was:

> Young ladies all, of every clime,
> Especially of Britain,
> Who wholly occupy your time
> In novels or in knitting
> Whose highest skill is but to play,
> Sing, dance, or French to clack well,
> Reflect on the example, pray,
> Of excellent Miss Blackwell!

After a warm welcome in London, Blackwell was crushed when French doctors dashed her hopes of studying in any Paris general hospital. Only one institution would accept her, an obstetrical hospital, La Maternité, where the twenty-eight-year-old American medical graduate, without rancor, willingly led the rigid life of an eighteen-year-old French student midwife. Making the best of the situation, she worked to improve her methods of delivering babies in a hospital where 3,000 babies were born annually.

In late 1849 Madame Charrier, who directed courses in midwifery, gave Elizabeth a token of her approval, a lithograph of an earlier Blackwell taken from a history of celebrated midwives. Dr. Blackwell was moved, but she had been even more elated earlier when Dr. Dubois, who had had her barred from L'Ecole de Médicine, had presented her with written approval of her accomplishments at La Maternité and suggested that she might well become the best obstetrician, male or female, in America.

Blackwell's medical career almost came to an end in 1849 when tragedy struck. Washing the eye of an infant afflicted with ophthalmalia, a drop of infected water splashed in her eye. Her biographer, Ishbel Ross, records that by evening, her eye was swollen shut. The senior intern, Dr. Hippolyte Blot, rushed her to the operating room. He may have been drawn to her romantically while exchanging lessons in science with her for lessons in English. He requested relief from his hospital duties entirely for a while to care for Dr. Blackwell. He confined her to bed in complete darkness, and steadily applied compresses. The only method known then were ineffective leechings, ointments, and compresses.

No known medical remedy could have saved the sight of the eye, and it had to be removed surgically.

Weeks later, when Elizabeth saw her reflection in the mirror for the first time after her illness, the full force of her disfigurement struck her and for the first time in her life, she became hysterical. Elizabeth's sister, Anna Blackwell, was working in Paris as a newspaper correspondent. While Elizabeth recuperated and adjusted to using one eye, she roomed with Anna. Elizabeth may have been in love with Blot. He had paid attention to her and had been especially kind. But now, with this handicap, she may have told him their friendship or courtship was over. Blackwell, usually so frank about her life, left no clue about her real feelings toward Dr. Blot.

Suddenly all the hospitals in Paris began issuing invitations to Blackwell to attend lectures and clinics. Unable to read with one eye and having lost her skill at dissection, she relinquished hope of being a surgeon. For her own mental health, she had to leave Paris. She visited Germany, and then returned to London to take lectures at St. Bartholomew's Hospital. She became a frequent guest at Brighton with Lady Byron, the widow of the famed poet. Sometimes Elizabeth walked with her friend, Florence Nightingale, around the magnificent estate of Embley. One day, in front of the manor, Florence put an arm around Elizabeth and remarked, "Do you know what I think when I look at that row of windows? I believe I should turn it into a hospital ward. I even know how I'd arrange the beds!"

Elizabeth remembered thinking that Florence's parents might not like that scheme. She was grateful for the social conscience of her own parents. At the time, Elizabeth could have no idea that Nightingale would eventually achieve world fame for her desire to make hospitals humane.

After two years of European postgraduate studies, Dr. Blackwell felt prepared to practice medicine in America. In 1851 she sailed for home, only to face seven hard years in New York.

Every previous challenge was dwarfed by these disappointing years. Landladies who had rooms for rent closed the door in her face when she admitted she wanted space for a clinic. She had to rent a whole floor, more than she could afford. Her landlady was outraged when Blackwell hung a small shingle. Few patients came, and they were reluctant to trust her. She was lonely because she had no one with whom to consult. When one of her patients had pneumonia, she called in a doctor who had cared for the patient's father in his final illness. The doctor, after examining the patient, silently walked with Blackwell to the living room, pacing in agitation. "A most extraordinary case. I really don't know what to do."

Dr. Blackwell was stunned. Clearly, pneumonia was not that unusual. Why was this man blowing it out of all proportion? Finally, the old man admitted his perplexity related to a woman doctor and not to the patient. He "couldn't determine the propriety of consulting with a lady physician." Blackwell hid her smile and reassured the old doctor that he could just regard the consultation as a friendly conversation. He proceeded to give her his best advice, which she took. The patient recovered.

From this experience, Blackwell learned how to talk with a male doctor. She never again had difficulty in obtaining consultations.

She requested a position in every hospital and dispensary in New York, but not one would consider her application. She was told to start her own dispensary, an idea she tucked away for further consideration. To occupy long empty hours in her office, she wrote a series of lectures and hired a hall. She advertised in the *Times*. Tickets were $2 for six lectures. Among her small audience were Quaker women who had long been discussing establishing a medical college for women. Impressed with Blackwell's ideas on room ventilation, exercise for girls, sensible nutrition, and comfortable clothing, the Quaker women became her patients. Her practice began to support her. She continued to have opposition from her male counterparts and from women too.

In 1858 Elizabeth and her sister, Emily, launched the New York Infirmary for Women and Children. Most medical schools had no entrance requirements or examinations, but from its beginning, the New York Infirmary required such examinations, a decade before they were compulsory elsewhere. The medical course, a graded curriculum, required three and a half years of intense work and studies. Elsewhere, medical students could complete their studies in two years with five months of instruction each year.

Blackwell created a chair of hygiene, which she filled. She established a visiting nurse service to city slums. Directed by Dr. Rebecca Cole, it became a model for the visiting nurse program in city slums everywhere. Dr. Cole, the second black woman to receive a medical degree in America, graduated from Woman's Medical College of Pennsylvania in 1867. (The first black woman to receive a medical degree may have been Rebecca Lee, who graduated from the New England Female Medical College, Boston, in 1864.)

When Fanny Kemble, the British actress, toured America in benefit performances, Blackwell recalled meeting the actress at Lord Byron's London home. Miss Kemble was known for her generosity in giving charity performances. Elizabeth approached her to do a performance for the benefit of her charity hospital. Kemble listened graciously until it dawned on her that the hospital was not only for women patients but also for women doctors! Her face reflected her disgust. "Trust a woman as a doctor!" Her voice rose dramatically, "Never! Never!"

Despite the discrimination with which she had to contend, Elizabeth never lost her sense of humor. She liked to tell a story about Kitty. To appease her great loneliness, in 1854 she adopted a seven-year-old orphan, Katherine Barrie. The girl brought great pleasure to Blackwell. Kitty called her "Doctor" rather than "Mother." During the visit of a consulting physician, Kitty seemed puzzled. After he left, she said to Blackwell, "Doctor, how very odd it is to hear a man called doctor!"

Marie Elizabeth Zakrzewska

In 1854 Elizabeth Blackwell's younger sister, Emily, followed in her footsteps, graduating from the medical school at Western Reserve University in Cleveland. The two sisters had long considered founding a hospital. With the appearance on the scene of a twenty-six-year-old Polish woman, the idea of a medical school for women became an obsession.

A large, unattractive woman with great energy, Marie Zakrzewska was born in Berlin in 1829. Her father, a Polish officer and patriot, had been exiled to Germany. The women in Marie's mother's family had a long tradition of midwifery. Her father encouraged Marie's career as a midwife. But to be a doctor? Never!

Marie persisted in her ambitions. By the time she was twenty-two, she was chief of the delivery room at Berlin's Charity Hospital and taught classes for up to 100 women and fifty men. In the hospital, Marie had to cope with resentment, rankling envy, and petty politics; she resigned after six months. Marie had met Elizabeth Blackwell in 1853 and became convinced that her future lay in America, where she would be a doctor.

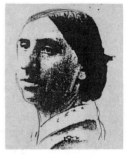

Of Marie Zakrzewska, Elizabeth Blackwell wrote to her sister Emily, "There is true stuff in her, and I shall do my best to bring it out. She must obtain a medical degree." *(Photo courtesy of New York Infirmary, 1901.)*

When Zakrzewska first arrived in New York, German doctors picked up on her father's belittling efforts to discourage her from her goal of becoming a doctor. "Take up nursing," they urged. Why was she surprised to learn that women physicians were regarded with little respect and were considered even inferior to nurses? To her, nursing was better than sewing, which was her means of earning a livelihood when she first settled in America.

Dr. Zak (as she was known from the time she despaired of teaching Americans to pronounce her name) came to America with halting English. Blackwell, speaking fluent German, welcomed her to the staff of her new dispensary. Zak proved herself a successful fund-raiser and repaid Blackwell's kindness by dedicated service for two years in the infirmary without salary.

Zak studied English and medical books and applied to the Cleveland Medical School. One of the first four women accepted in 1854, she finally achieved her cherished goal and graduated with an M.D. in 1856.

With the outbreak of the Civil War, Dr. Zak and Emily and Elizabeth Blackwell directed their energies to helping women get accepted by medical organizations and to training nurses.

Dr. Zak was resident physician of the New York Infirmary from 1857 to 1859, when the New England Female Medical College invited her to become its first professor in obstetrics. The college shut down its hospital, and Dr. Zak helped organize what became known as the New England Hospital, the first in America with a nursing school. In this hospital for women and children, Zak, brilliant and creative, started a social services program and won recognition as one of Boston's leading physicians. Eventually, she retired to a country home that became a social center for her German and American friends. She died in 1902.

Dorothea Lynde Dix

Civil War nurse, teacher, social reformer, and philanthropist Dorothea Dix, a remarkably intrepid Victorian woman, became famous for her compassion and concern for inmates of mental asylums.

Born in Hampden, Maine, in 1802, she was reared by an extremely religious father, Joseph Dix. Harvard-educated, a pulpit orator, and an author, he taught his daughter the Bible and the classics. When she was thirteen, he ordered her to help his holy mission. Dorothea rebelled and ran away to her widowed grandmother in Boston. Though surrounded by elegant antiques and bookshelves lined with leatherbound volumes, Dorothea could not abide her grandmother's rigidity. Worcester relatives invited her to live with them, and an uncle encouraged her to open a babysitting school in a building he owned. Teaching required no special qualifications, and at fourteen Dorothea relished being in charge. At sixteen, she returned to her parents and assumed the responsibility for both of her younger brothers.

Later, she became a governess and teacher with a family who invited her to join their voyage to the Caribbean. On a St. Croix plantation, eager to enlarge her scientific knowledge, she compiled long lists of wild and cultivated flora of the lovely tropical island. She seemed oblivious to the cruelty and inhumanity of slavery, which troubled her less than drunkenness. She talked to slaves and described their graceful figures. She thought they were more handsome than the whites. She envied what she considered the happiness of the children but was deeply troubled by the exploitation of enslaved women and the racially mixed offspring of white masters and black slaves. What troubled her most was the promiscuity involved.

In 1821 on her return to Boston, Dix opened her own school. By 1824 she had published a science textbook, *Conversations in Common Things*, which reached an astounding sixtieth edition by 1869. She edited *Hymns for Children and Evening Hours* in 1825, *Meditations for Private Hours* in 1828, and *Garland of Flora* in 1829.

Though she won the respect of many men, Dorothea seemed remarkably immune to romance. One of her students, Mary Eustis Channing, later recalled Dorothea's lockstep discipline as strict and inflexible. Dix continued teaching and writing until 1836, when tuberculosis forced her to abandon her school. She left Boston for England, where she spent two years. Still an invalid when she returned home, she was astounded to learn she had an inheritance that would support her for the rest of her life.

In 1841 a clergyman asked her to teach a Sunday school class in a prison. She was eager to do so, but was horrified at the treatment of the insane men and women who were housed with hardened criminals. Some were naked, some raving, all in terrible unsanitary conditions. She witnessed the flogging of inmates and poor wretches chained to walls. The experience changed her life. Determined to study other institutions for the insane, she traveled widely for two years, observing the horror of jails and almshouses. The first American to demand that the government assume responsibility for caring for insane paupers, she delivered her courageous message in the corridors of power. She waged an international crusade to reform the treatment of the mentally ill from Washington to Rome.

Profoundly religious, Dix was determined to fulfill God's call to speak for the mad. It was not her father's influence but Florence Nightingale's that inspired Dix's crusade. Determined to meet and even emulate Nightingale, in 1856 Dix sailed for Constantinople. There she was appalled by the dark terrors of the prisons and hospitals. Shivering in her shoes, she courageously hired a rowboat to cross the Bosporus to Scutari. Although Dix never met Nightingale, she was inspired by the English woman's success in transforming a miserable infirmary into a military hospital that became a therapeutic asylum.

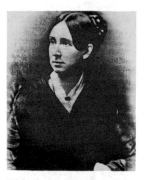

With a good education and close connections with Boston's intellectual circle, Dix urged the government to finance asylums for the mentally ill. *(Photo courtesy of Macmillan Books, 1910.)*

In 1844 Dix shifted from dramatizing the plight of the insane to influencing men of wealth and power to contribute to hospital construction. She persuaded a Rhode Island millionaire to donate $50,000 to enlarge what became the Butler Hospital for the Insane in Providence, an exceptional moment in the state's philanthropic history. During the following forty years, thirty-two institutions were built in the United States. Dix was responsible for legislation in fifteen American states and in Canada that established public institutions for the insane. On a tour of Europe in 1854–1856, she arranged a meeting with Pope Pius IX to urge him to inspect the terrible institutions she had seen.

Her book, *Remarks on Prisons and Prison Discipline in the United States,* published in 1845, brought about remarkable reforms in the treatment of the incarcerated.

During the Civil War, Dix saw a chance to lead a crusade. She would volunteer and willingly work without a salary, if she were granted responsibility to select and assign women nurses to military hospitals. She demanded a special title: superintendent of women nurses. Administrative leadership was sorely needed. Tough, blunt, demanding, and undiplomatic, Dix campaigned for decent care of the wounded with the same obsession she used to fight for humane care for the insane. She volunteered her services to organize, under the official auspices of the War Department, an Army Nursing Corps made up of volunteers. She was appointed but seemed more concerned with the morals of the nurses than with their training. In a letter to a friend, Louisa Lee Schuyler, Dix specified that "no woman under 30 need apply to serve in government hospitals. All nurses would be plain looking women. Their dresses had to be brown or black, with no bows, no curls, no jewelry, and no hoop-skirts."

Elizabeth Blackwell found Dix overbearing and dictatorial. A nurse called her "Dragon Dix." Another spoke of her as queer and arbitrary. Dix, too unbending to be a good administrator, alienated others who were more adept at administrative leadership. Her compassionate humanitarian Civil War missions carried out with determined courage deserve to be remembered and honored. After the war, she rededicated herself to working with the mentally ill. She died in 1887.

Elizabeth Garrett Anderson

In 1859 Elizabeth Garrett was in a large audience at Marylebone Institute in London listening intently to a lecture by Elizabeth Blackwell. The American doctor contrasted the dedicated service of French nuns with the useless life of ladies of leisure. Having a valuable role in life appealed to Elizabeth Garrett. She was moved by Blackwell's descriptions of the need for educated women to be well qualified as doctors, to serve other women and children, to teach mothers about nutrition and child rearing, and to make schools, prisons, and hospitals more humane.

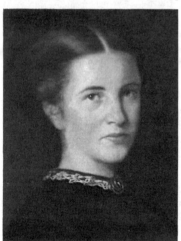

Elizabeth Garrett, c. 1860, earned her M.D. from the Sorbonne. *(Photo courtesy of Faber & Faber Ltd.)*

Garrett knew that British hospitals attempted to serve the worthy poor, the aged, the abandoned, the unemployed, and the terminally ill. Patients had to be sick to be admitted to the hospital, but ordinarily they also had to be indigent. Too frequently patients were treated with "a combination of condescension, contempt, and concern by trustees, physicians, and investigators who interviewed them at home before admission to evaluate their medical needs and moral environment."

At dinner, Garrett's father read aloud the observations of a newspaper columnist: "It is impossible that Dr. Blackwell, whose hands reek with gore, can be possessed of the same nature or feelings as the generality of women." Miss Garrett quickly defended Dr. Blackwell and added that she admired the American doctor.

Her father's business partner interposed that he was acquainted with the American doctor, and he offered a letter of introduction to "Miss Dr. Blackwell" for Garrett. When the two Elizabeths met face-to-face, Dr. Blackwell assumed she was speaking to a future colleague. Though Garrett felt she had no particular genius for medicine or anything else, the desire for a career in medicine was planted in her soul.

In the following weeks, with her good friend Emily Davies, she continued to attend Blackwell's lectures. Davies, obsessed with the need for women doctors, considered her intelligent friend the perfect medical pioneer.

In 1860 in *The Englishwoman's Journal*, Garrett read a letter from Dr. Blackwell describing a four-year medical course. Thinking constantly about medical school, she wondered if she could qualify for medicine in America or in Switzerland, where such schools were accepting women. But graduating from a foreign medical school would not qualify her to legally practice in England. She was determined to gain admission to a British medical school.

"Vested interest, prejudice, and custom, so potent in British society, were all against her," according to Jo Manton, Garrett's biographer. "Nowhere in Europe was the woman who wished to study medicine so stubbornly opposed as in Britain, yet nowhere was her final victory so complete." Among the many reasons for Elizabeth's victory was the strength of her character; she was the first English woman to qualify as a physician and surgeon.

Garrett plunged into studies with tutors. Her father, who had recently recovered from financial setbacks, made it clear to his twenty-four-year-old daughter that the very idea she wanted to be a doctor was disgusting.

This opposition only stiffened Garrett's resolve. The Newson Garretts had four sons and six daughters. If a brother had announced his intent to become a doctor, he would have been praised and assisted. "What is there to make doctoring more disgusting than nursing, which women are always doing . . . which ladies have done in the Crimea?" Elizabeth wondered.

Her father warned her she would be committed to seven years of hard study before she could practice medicine. Elizabeth countered, "Six, not seven; and if it were seven years, I should be little more than 31 years old and able to work for 20 years probably."

Later, at a dinner party, Garrett had the satisfaction of overhearing her father say he would actually prefer a woman doctor for his wife and daughters. Elizabeth had won her father's admiring support, but not her mother's. Mrs. Garrett, with ten children, was unstrung by her daughter's decision to study medicine. If Elizabeth needed to be useful, why not stay home and take care of her younger siblings? For Elizabeth, this suggestion had all the charm of cold mashed potatoes. Why couldn't her mother understand that Elizabeth did not want to spend the rest of her life in the Garrett home?

The daughter asked her father to introduce her to some of his doctor friends on Harley Street. Though the physicians were gracious, they pointed to the Medical Act of 1858, which clearly stated that to be enrolled on the Medical Register required licensing by a qualified examining board of a British university. No British examining board had ever admitted a woman. "Why not be a nurse?" Elizabeth replied emotionally, "Because I prefer to earn a thousand rather than twenty pounds a year."

Though her father admired her spirit, Elizabeth worried he would learn about the demand for women to be nurses. A nurses' training school, endowed by the Nightingale Fund, was opening at St. Thomas's Hospital, and "lady pupils" were urged to take hospital training. Miss Garrett rejected the idea that women's nursing should complement men's medical careers.

In 1860 Garrett, through friends of Elizabeth Blackwell, the Russell Gurneys, met a director of Middlesex Hospital who urged her to do a six-month "trial marriage at the hospital, simply working as a nurse." Garrett accepted the challenge at what was then London's finest teaching hospital. Although many medical students have nightmares about anatomy and surgery, Garrett faced the ordeal of the surgical ward with calm resolve. Maintaining a healthy detachment, she prepared poultices and ointments, rolled bandages, and dressed wounds. She prudently kept her medical ambitions to herself, accompanying a head nurse and observing closely. The house surgeons were helpful to her after Dr. T. W. Nunn made a point of explaining a ward operation, and Nunn pleased her by inviting her to his outpatient clinics.

She regarded the long whitewashed walls, rows of curtained beds, and bare floors as dehumanizing. Middlesex surgeons wore old frocks in dissecting and operating rooms until the coats, stiffened with blood and pus, stood upright. The operating assistants, like angels hovering above a doomed crib, circled the wood table, bloody as a butcher's block, and contributed their germs to those of the pushing and jostling student throng. Sometimes the odors made her sick. Gangrene could be carried from patient to patient by the nurses.

Garrett completed her six-month probation at Middlesex Hospital and abandoned the pretense of being a nurse. As an unofficial medical student, she made rounds in wards, worked in the dispensary, helped with emergency patients, and studied with private tutors. In December her examinations covering the work of the previous five months impressed her teachers.

No British university had ever accepted a woman. Would Oxford or Cambridge change the rules to admit Elizabeth Garrett? Her father discussed with her the charter of the University of London: "All persons" who fulfilled the requirements would be admitted to the examinations, and "denominations without distinction" would be admitted. Now fiercely determined to help his daughter, Mr. Garrett insisted that "persons" be regarded as including women. His daughter must be allowed to take the examinations.

The Society of Apothecaries in London was willing to examine her knowledge if she could fulfill the regulations, which included three years in a British medical school. By this time, she had a certificate from Dr. Joshua Plaskitt showing a successful apprenticeship. Some university might accept her. She applied to St. Andrews in Scotland. At the time, students were required only to buy "matriculation" tickets for one pound. When functionaries at St. Andrews discovered that Garrett had bought a ticket for a lecture series to which she'd been invited by a professor, the school refunded her money with a sharp request that the ticket be returned. Elizabeth Garrett threatened to sue.

Rejected by St. Andrews, Garrett tried Edinburgh University, and was promptly rejected. Again, Garrett turned to private tutoring, this time in Edinburgh with Dr. Stevenson Macadam and the famous Sir James Young Simpson, who had previously tutored Elizabeth and Emily Blackwell.

Garrett was fortunate to study midwifery with Dr. Alexander Keiller at the Edinburgh Maternity Hospital, where he had established the first systematic clinical teaching in gynecology. She also studied for a year at the Royal Maternity with a surgeon, Dr. David Murray, who reported twenty-five cases of successful vaccination of the newborn, a subject in which Garrett retained a lifelong interest. Every delivery of a healthy baby thrilled her. "I wonder," she wrote, "if one will go on feeling an immediate affection for the little creatures that come first into your hands. I did everything a doctor does usually and found it very easy."

Back in London, Garrett applied again to take the examinations of the Society of Apothecaries. She was overjoyed to be accepted. But her happiness was cut short when she received a letter from the school reneging at the last moment. The authorities told her to try again in five years. Perhaps they suspected that such a lovely woman would be married in half a decade with a few children underfoot. Incensed, Newson Garrett issued an ultimatum, threatening a lawsuit if Elizabeth were not admitted to take the examinations. Angrily, he stressed that the charter of the school did not exclude women.

At last she was summoned to come for the examinations. She found them incredibly easy. No written papers or clinical trials were required. She sailed through the questions on medicine, midwifery, and pathology and became one of only three candidates to receive a final certificate.

Now with the degree of Licentiate of the Society of Apothecaries (LSA), she was entitled to be admitted to the Medical Register. The LSA was not as prestigious as an M.D., but it allowed her to practice medicine in England.

Mr. Garrett rented and generously furnished a modest office for her. He himself hung the small shingle that said "Elizabeth Garrett, LSA." In addition to her private practice, she started a small clinic, St. Mary's Dispensary for Women. Within weeks of its opening in a slum, she was examining and treating as many as a hundred women. A few years later, the dispensary grew into the New Hospital for Women.

Community medicine for women and children was a crying need. Garrett was more than a doctor; she was also a pharmacist, surgeon, nurse, and counselor to the poor. Stories told by her victimized, dirt-poor patients thrust her into the women's rights movement.

Garrett felt discriminated against because she had so few doctors with whom she could consult. She longed to be on the consulting staff of a good hospital, preferably Shadwell Hospital for Children. Never having used feminine wiles to achieve a goal, she debated about relaxing this once. She applied to the board of the Shadwell Hospital, and at the next meeting met a bachelor who confessed he strongly opposed admitting a woman to the consulting staff. He added that he thought she was very beautiful. Lowering her eyes, Garrett replied demurely. She received the appointment.

When patients addressed her as "Doctor," she corrected them, saying she had never earned an M.D. and would not take credit for something she did not have. She had certainly achieved a hard-won practice, but she was determined to earn an M.D., something she could not achieve in England. She would follow Elizabeth Blackwell's example and go to the University of Paris, which granted medical degrees to women. Would the British ambassador arrange for her to take entrance examinations in Paris? Lord Lyons agreed to try. Not long afterward, Garrett received permission to sit for the medical examinations. Though she had studied French in school, she had long ago forgotten most of it.

In Paris at thirty-two, Garrett awoke with the sun and studied French verbs and chemistry. Mary Putnam, the American graduate of Woman's Medical College in Philadelphia, had been working in Paris hospitals since 1866. After eighteen months of constant refusals to the medical faculty on grounds that no woman had ever been accepted, Putnam was admitted at last in 1868. All Garrett wanted was permission to take six examinations required for a medical degree in France.

The name of Elizabeth Garrett was familiar to the French because of the publicity surrounding her refusals at St. Andrews. The French dean of the Faculty of Medicine supported her, but applications for admission had come at the same time from two other foreign women, and the rest of the faculty feared an influx of women. Garrett was again rejected.

However, Lord Lyons, a diplomatic friend of France, had promised to help Garrett's cause and prevailed upon Empress Eugenie to intervene and authorize the admission of all three women applicants. In February 1869, a letter informed Lord Lyons that Garrett could come the following month to take her first examination in Paris.

She faced three examiners in black robes. Behind her sat male students and lecturers on tiers of benches almost to the roof. With a pounding heart, she responded to questions so well that the gallery broke into applause.

In June 1869, her second examination required her to perform two surgical procedures in the presence of judges and medical students. She wrote her thesis on headaches, the pathology of migraine.

In December she took the third M.D. examination in Paris: chemistry, philosophy (physics), zoology, and botany, and passed with *bien satisfait,* the highest grade possible in these subjects. On December 24, she again faced three examiners, this time in medical jurisprudence, hygiene, and *materia medica.* On January 4 she took her fifth and final examination in clinical medicine, midwifery, and surgery. At long last, in June, in a long black wool gown, she read her thesis aloud and defended it to the questioners. When she finished reading, the candidate and the spectators left the room while the judges deliberated. She returned to be congratulated as the first woman M.D. of the Sorbonne!

Even the *British Medical Journal,* still hostile to women in medicine, expressed admiration for the "perseverance and pluck which Miss Garrett has shown." (They did not have the courtesy to call her "Dr. Garrett.") A headline in *The Times* (London), March 22, 1870, announced, "Miss Garrett admitted on a Regular Medical Staff."

When Garrett had opened her dispensary in 1866, she was thirty years old and had the assistance of Dr. Nathaniel Heckford during a cholera epidemic. Now Dr. Heckford hoped to open a children's hospital in East London. After some opposition from the board, including a hesitant James George Skelton Anderson who was personally attracted to the lovely doctor, Garrett was named medical officer.

Taking up her duties at the East London Hospital in 1870, Dr. Garrett cared for women and children. Working men of the district asked her to run for the school board. For the first time ever, the community was to have free compulsory education. She could not refuse and was overwhelmingly elected. James Anderson hurried to congratulate her on her victory and, as if in afterthought, asked Elizabeth to marry him. She did not hesitate. She loved him. Of course she would marry him.

Garrett's acceptance puzzled her father. After having expended so much money, effort, and sheer gall to get her degree, why would she throw over a career for marriage? His daughter replied she had no intention of giving up her medical practice. James Anderson may have had to hide his surprise at first, but he became supportive of his wife's combining marriage with a successful medical career.

From 1874 to 1878, medical education for women became secured. Elizabeth Garrett lectured at the London School of Medicine for Women and continued to work for education for the rest of her life.

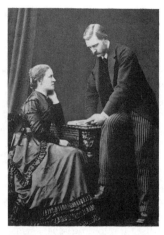

Elizabeth Garrett and James Anderson in their engagement portrait. *(Photo courtesy of Faber & Faber.)*

In 1874 the London School of Medicine enrolled fourteen women. A quarter of a century passed before women, in 1896, could win the privilege of residency at Royal Free Hospital. That year, the Royal College of Physiology in Ireland and London University admitted women to examinations to qualify for a medical career. These graduates established practices, but often could not find a male doctor willing to consult with them. For a long time, women were prohibited from joining medical societies.

Sometime around 1880, the wife of an Indian barrister and the mother of two children, Mary Scharlieb, came to Dr. Garrett. Having seen the suffering of women in purdah who had no prenatal or childbirth care, Mary Scharlieb had trained at Madras for the Indian Medical Practitioners Certificate. Now she wanted to study at the London School of Medicine for Women. Dr. Garrett helped her enroll and recognized in her the potential of a gifted surgeon. Scharlieb took honors and a gold medal in obstetrics.

By 1883 Elizabeth was elected dean of the London School of Medicine. Her first official duty was to present Mary Scharlieb and another graduating student, Edith Shove, to Lord Granville, the chancellor, for graduation. Twenty-one years had passed since Lord Granville's vote had been instrumental in refusing Garrett's petition to be examined by the university. It seemed appropriate to Dr. Garrett Anderson to write her father, asking him to come for the graduation exercises. Grey bearded, Newson Garrett, in frock coat, watched the chancellor, in full academic dress, hand scrolls to the candidates.

Before Scharlieb returned to India with her husband, she was summoned by Queen Victoria, who exclaimed, "How can they tell me there is no need for medical women in India? Tell them how deeply their Queen sympathizes with them and how glad she is that they should have medical women to help them in their time of need."

Elizabeth and James Anderson had a happy marriage and two children. In 1902 they moved to Aldeburgh to the lovely old home Mr. Garrett left to his favorite daughter. James Anderson was elected mayor of Aldeburgh, and when he died in 1907, Elizabeth was asked to complete his term. In the following election, she was returned to office in her own right, the first woman mayor ever elected in England.

Her daughter, Louisa, from the time she was a child, knew she would be a doctor like her mother. Elizabeth Garrett Anderson died at eighty-one, in 1917. The New Hospital for Women, recognized and respected throughout the medical world, was renamed the Elizabeth Garrett Anderson Hospital in her honor.

Sophia Jex-Blake

Elizabeth Garrett Anderson, a standard-bearer for women in Victorian society, earned a medical degree through a series of small skirmishes. What about other women who wanted to be doctors? The battle was begun. Sophia Jex-Blake turned it into a full-scale war.

In Edinburgh in 1862, Sophia Jex-Blake's imagination was fired by Garrett's efforts to apply for admission to medical school. She had insisted on going with Garrett to the interview. Brashly, Jex-Blake put in her two cents. The Edinburgh medical faculty assumed that the gentle, sweet Garrett sitting beside the brash Sophia Jex-Blake was there to support the sharp-tongued woman. But Sophia, with her flashing dark eyes and aggressive manners, had her own agenda: reforming education for women. She had just completed a miserable year of teaching English to rambunctious German girls in a school in Mannheim. She was determined to escape from her father's authority and sail for the United States to study colleges and to write a book about American higher education.

Sophia Jex-Blake, born in Hastings, Sussex, in 1840, had graduated from Queen's College for Women, in London. There may be some correlation between a sour, ultraconservative father and the proud achievements of a rebellious daughter. Perhaps in the girl's mind, a defiance grows that stimulates her somehow to accomplish what her parent insists can't be done. Every pressure put on Sophia to turn a bright, energetic, innovative girl into a dutiful daughter only made her more stubborn and independent. Pursuing an education, she found what was offered to women stultifying. Many a young woman marries just to escape from a home where parents disapprove of her goals or attitudes. Sophia, at eighteen, had no desire to be married. Learning that Queen's College had opened for women, she made up her mind to enroll, but she had to engage in hysterics before her father would permit her to go.

Within a few months after winning the heady freedom of campus life, Sophia began to tutor math. Her father wrote her that it was demeaning for her to accept pay for tutoring, and he urged her to teach as a volunteer. Sophia, excited about earning her own living, ignored his advice.

In 1866 Jex-Blake arrived in Boston with a letter of introduction for Dr. Lucy Sewall, a colleague of Marie Zakrzewska at the New England Hospital for Women. Dr. Sewall, peering at Jex-Blake through terrible spectacles that magnified the entire eyeball, assigned Sophia to work in the dispensary. Jex-Blake discovered her natural talent for administration. She was thrilled by the companionship of professional women who delivered babies, bravely performed surgery, and managed their own hospital. "Besides being an apothecary," she wrote home, "I'm general secretary . . . and put up the hospital records of cases, etc."

In 1866 she applied to Harvard and received a form letter rejecting her. She had brought with her a letter to Elizabeth and Emily Blackwell. Sophia, learning that the sisters had opened their medical school, became their fiery, enthusiastic first student.

She had been in America three years, pursuing medical courses and writing a book on higher education in America, when her father's final illness called her home. After his death, she returned to Edinburgh where she had supported Elizabeth Garrett's appeals for admission to the medical school. Ironically, though most of Jex-Blake's friends encouraged her, Dr. Garrett did not. Garrett had learned through tough experience that medicine requires objectivity, and she considered Jex-Blake's drawbacks: temperament, intense loves and hates, and sensitivity to criticism. She told Jex-Blake, "Frankly, I think you're not specially suited." Garrett was not alone in this opinion; many people found Jex-Blake irritating.

Initially, Jex-Blake approached two influential men at Edinburgh who might help her, David Masson of the university English Department and the invaluable Sir James Simpson. Sir James arranged a meeting with the dean of the Medical School, Dr. Balfour. The dean, attempting to be sympathetic, pointed out she would be required to dissect a cadaver. Jex-Blake assured him that she had already dissected several cadavers in America. Dr. Balfour knew she had proven abilities as a scholar with a published book on higher education in the United States. He could permit her to enroll for two summer courses, botany and natural history. Jex-Blake was satisfied to be accepted to the college, even though it was "the edge of the wedge," as she described it.

A few weeks later, she received a letter from the authorities reneging on the permission because this temporary arrangement in the interest of only one "lady," was too difficult for the university to work out.

Only one lady! What a challenge! Within two months, Jex-Blake returned, slyly admitting the authorities were right. It would hardly be worthwhile to change the rules for only one woman. She had with her four women, and all five applied for admission, with two more planning to apply the following year.

Jex-Blake recruited these women, who volunteered partly to help her, because she had been rebuffed as the solitary applicant. Among these recruits was Isobel Thorne, a married woman who had witnessed appalling health conditions in China and British indifference to them. Thorne had considered studying medicine, and the publicity surrounding Jex-Blake convinced her to apply to Edinburgh University. The other applicants, Edith Pechey, twenty-four years old, full of self-doubt, was pushed by Jex-Blake, and Helen Evans and Matilda Chaplin made up the "gallant little band." Jex-Blake proposed that the university permit her and the four women to take entrance examinations and register to study for a medical degree. She made the mistake of guaranteeing that extra fees could be paid to compensate for any separate accommodations necessary for teaching women. After considerable legislating, Edinburgh, for the first time in its history, enrolled women as students in a British university. However, they were required to pay three times as much as male undergraduates.

All went smoothly, and although the women were taught in classes separate from the men, they studied the same subjects. The honeymoon ended when grades were published, causing keen embarrassment to a faculty that had long maintained that women had smaller, inferior brains. Of 140 male students, 32 had taken honors in botany. All five women took honors. In chemistry, 32 of 226 men took honors. Four of the five women students also took honors. One woman, gentle Edith Pechey, who worried she might be unable to compete with the men, won top class honors in chemistry and walked away with the coveted Hope Scholarship. She was excused from paying laboratory fees the following year.

Edinburgh admitted the five women, expecting them to be unable to cope with the strenuous program. Now the chemistry professor, Dr. Crum Brown, handed Edith Pechey's prize to the male student just below her, because Pechey was not a regular class member and so was ineligible for the prize. When this news appeared in the British press, the Scots were up in arms. In the past, the five women had been regarded as eccentrics, but now all Edinburgh waxed indignant in letters to the editor.

That summer, two new recruits joined the five women at Edinburgh, and in historic Surgeons' Hall, two sympathetic professors taught anatomy and surgery to seven women in an academic atmosphere. In November, when the women were to take examinations in anatomy, Jex-Blake and her fellow students were mobbed as they tried to enter Surgeons' Hall. The police ignored the situation as gates were slammed in the women's faces. Students, vagrants, and toughs screamed insults at them. Finally a classmate ran down to open the door of the hall and pull open the gates, ushering the women to their class. All through the examination, the mob outside hooted, howled, and cursed.

When the session was complete, a professor suggested the women might like to leave through the rear entrance. Jex-Blake, furious, thanked him and assured him there were probably some gentlemen in the class to help the women get safely home. Four young men escorted the women through the mob that still waited, pelting the women students with mud and insults. In this threatening atmosphere, Edinburgh citizens formed a Committee to Secure Complete Medical Education to Women in Edinburgh. At a mass meeting supporting the rights of women to study medicine, a grandmother rose to ask, "If students studying in the Infirmary cannot accept women as fellow students, how can they have the scientific spirit or personal purity of mind to justify their presence in female wards during delicate operations or examinations of female patients?" Hoots, howls, and hisses came from the balcony. When Jex-Blake attempted to speak, she was hit with spitballs. The horseplay was so loud she couldn't be heard.

A group of Irish students began escorting the women to and from class until the mob lost interest. Sophia expressed gratitude to one of the men, who suggested the women should have gone to school in Ireland where they would never have had anything but courtesy. "I remembered his words," Jex-Blake wrote later, "when in 1876, the Irish College of Physicians was the first of all the Examining Boards to admit women."

The Edinburgh faculty, even those who had been friendly and supportive to the women, were now intimidated by Jex-Blake's enemies and refused to arrange for private tutoring for the few remaining courses needed for the women's graduation. Not even the smallest concession could be made to arrange for helping them get a medical degree. On the contrary, the university offered certificates of proficiency as an alternative. Jex-Blake angrily insisted that the university had allowed women to begin their medical studies and to continue them at great expense. She turned to the law.

The courts found for Jex-Blake and the women students. The university was now bound in justice to provide a way for their studies to be completed. Not only were the women allowed to continue classes, but they could also at long last do clinical work at the Royal Infirmary.

Jex-Blake, involved in litigation and committee work, was close to exhaustion when she took her final examinations. For the rest of her life, she would be haunted by the results. She was the only one of the women medical students who failed. At the same time, the lower court's decision finding in favor of the women medical students was reversed; the judges declared that the University of Edinburgh was not obligated to let the women graduate because the powers of the university had been exceeded by admitting women in the first place.

The court rubbed salt in their wounds by saddling the women with the costs of both hearings, although it had specified that the university had been in error in 1869 when they were admitted.

After four long years of strenuous study and struggle, Sophia Jex-Blake and her companions were no nearer to the Medical Register than they had been in 1869. Jex-Blake had become notorious.

Jex-Blake later maintained that her finals had not been poor enough to justify failing grades. "The faculty had failed her out of spite." An article in the *Times* commented that it was amusing that "one of the ladies who had rendered herself most conspicuous should after all have failed under the test of examinations."

Jex-Blake made up her mind to start her own hospital. She found a house; directed the builders painters, and plumbers; and did what she was best at—administration. She signed up a teaching staff and registered a dozen students. In 1874 her London School of Medicine for Women opened its doors.

Two years later, with the London School running smoothly, Jex-Blake and Edith Pechey went to Bern to fulfill the hours of hospital and clinical studies and take university examinations required by Switzerland to qualify them to write "M.D." after their names. Eight years had passed since the time they should have had that distinction and that right. The year 1876 remains a milestone, not only in the life of Sophia Jex-Blake, but in the history of education and medicine for women. That year a bill was passed in England enabling all universities of the United Kingdom and Ireland to grant degrees to women. The bill owes not a little to the spunk and stamina of outspoken Sophia Jex-Blake.

She was thirty-six the year she studied at Bern to prepare for medical examinations, and she was not without qualms that she might fail. She passed. That evening, she wrote in her diary: "Now to see how much better an M.D. sleeps than other people!"

Jex-Blake and Pechey still had to take licensing examinations in Dublin. On May 6, 1877, two successful women candidates were licensed to practice as members of the Irish College of Physicians. Their names, entered on the Medical Register of England, opened the way for all qualified women doctors. They had won for women the right to a medical education, to hospital residencies, and to inclusion in the Medical Register.

Bursting with triumphant energy, Jex-Blake returned to the London School of Medicine she had founded. The Royal Free Hospital of London had agreed to admit women for clinical training—providing they paid fees to subsidize the hospital. An executive secretary was to be appointed, and Dr. Jex-Blake was qualified for this honorary position. However, in her absence, a group opposed to her nominated Elizabeth Garrett Anderson. Garrett refused the honor, but she suggested Isobel Thorne as an alternative. Dr. Thorne accepted the position and proved to be a capable, tactful administrator for thirty years. Jex-Blake respected her, but felt justly deprived that the school she had founded was run by someone else. Heavyhearted, she left London to return to Edinburgh.

In 1885 Jex-Blake launched a hospital in Edinburgh for needy women and children. The hospital faithfully served the city that was witness to a great women's crusade.

The demands of Jex-Blake for justice won her the reputation of a battle-ax. Demands for justice usually come from angry, morally indignant people. To exclude anger from human communication, as Rousseau observed, is to concentrate all passion in a "self-interest of the meanest sort." Such a universe would offer no progress. Sophia Jex-Blake's book, *Medical Women*, published in 1886, was among the first on a subject that changed attitudes about women's roles in the world.

Mary Putnam Jacobi

Mary Corinna Putnam, the eldest of ten children, born in London, England, in 1842, was educated at home, with special studies in anatomy. Her father, George Palmer Putnam, founder of a famous New York publishing house, endowed his favorite daughter with a love for science as well as his for literature.

When she was seventeen, Mary was thrilled and surprised that her first story, "Lost and Found," sold to the *Atlantic Monthly*. Her father got hold of the check and proudly converted it into five-dollar gold pieces that he dropped one by one into Mary's hand. With each piece, she squealed. Eighty dollars! That was a fortune in those days.

Had Mary Putnam decided on pursuing literature rather than medicine as a career, she might have been among the famous authors of nineteenth-century America. Instead, she gained admission as its first woman student to the New

York College of Pharmacy and graduated in 1863. Mary Putnam hoped the pharmacy degree would be a stepping-stone toward a medical career. Her supportive father wrote her he was proud of her abilities and "willing that she should apply them even to the repulsive pursuit of medical education." He urged her to preserve her feminine character and "the elegances of life."

She was twenty-one when she left New York to enroll in the Female Medical College in Philadelphia, the first such college in the world. Dr. Ann Preston (1813–1872), a courageous Quaker, directed the college, founded in 1850. During the Civil War, the college shared the fate of others and closed for lack of financial support. After the war, Dr. Preston reopened the college and resumed her efforts to get the women graduates accepted in medical organizations.

Elizabeth Blackwell recorded her impressions of Ann Preston: "fragile . . . a delicate, refined Quaker lady . . . who came to me out of the wild snow storm . . . I was sure that she would succeed."

Ann Preston, a professor of physiology, successfully enrolled students at Pennsylvania Hospital. But they were greeted with "jeers, groaning, whistling, and foot stamping" by the men students. "On leaving the hospital, we were actually stoned by the so-called gentlemen," one student, Elizabeth Keller, remembered. She persisted and graduated to become chief of surgery at the New England Hospital for Women and Children.

When Mary Putnam looked over the two-year course of study at the Female Medical College, she realized that the same sets of lectures were offered each year, the second year being merely a repetition of the first. Determined not to miss a lecture, Putnam made up her mind to take the examinations at the end of the year. Her studies in pharmacy helped her to pass with flying colors. In 1864 Mary and six classmates received medical degrees in a dreary waiting room of the Women's Hospital. She interned at New England Hospital for Women in Boston, founded two years earlier by the well-known "Dr. Zak, Marie Zakrzewska."

When Mary completed her internship, she needed a qualified tutor and recalled a gifted young German scientist, Ferdinand Mayer, who had taught chemistry at the College of Pharmacy. Mary's father questioned whether his daughter should be alone in a laboratory with the professor. Mr. Putnam suggested his second son take up chemistry. The boy agreed and learned a little science while he acted as chaperone, oblivious to a growing affection between his sister and Professor Mayer.

Mary's mother announced her eldest daughter's engagement to Dr. Mayer. As the September wedding day drew near, Mary wavered and began to consider marriage to Dr. Mayer a mistake. Strong-minded Mary Putnam broke her engagement.

Dissatisfied with her education in medicine, she thought American doctors relied too much on observation and experience. They often scorned microscopes and stethoscopes. What she longed to do was go to Europe to continue her medical education. How to pay for it? G. P. Putnam publishing house had suffered a financial crisis, and Mary hardly covered expenses in her medical practice. To finance her European studies, Mary tutored a young man who wanted to pass West Point entrance examinations. In 1866 when Mary's pupil successfully passed the test, Putnam's brother observed wryly, "After a year of working with a slave driver like Mary, the young man may find West Point discipline a relief!" Years later, Dr. Putnam's students at Woman's Medical College complained about what they regarded as her unreasonable expectations.

With funds from her tutoring, Mary arrived in France without knowing a word of French. She enrolled in the University of Paris anyway. Thanks to Elizabeth Blackwell, who was in France at the time, Mary was able to rent a room with a view so lovely she remembered it with joy for the rest of her life. Within months, Mary Putnam was conversing in French, although her accent had her French listeners covering their ears in distress.

She began working in hospitals and was soon respected for her competence at diagnosis. A day before making rounds with the doctors, she would examine patients and question them. One day at Beaujon, a doctor asked her if she agreed with another physician's diagnosis of typhoid.

"No, Monsieur, it's mumps!" Putnam replied with confidence. She then offered corroboration for her diagnosis.

"Correct!" exclaimed the doctor. Turning to the other medical students, he said, "Gentlemen, good students are not afraid to offer a minor ailment as a diagnosis."

The first time she used a microscope her heart beat so hard she could hear the pounding in her ears. She observed surgery in the clinic and studied in the medical library.

The French minister of public instruction was progressive and willing to have women admitted to the medical school. Dr. Putnam made a formal application to the school but no one in the admissions office seemed to have heard of the progressive minister's views. Dr. Putnam was promptly refused.

Her disappointment, however, was assuaged by a professor of histology, who welcomed her to his lectures. For the first time since the school's founding centuries earlier, students became accustomed to seeing an attractive woman taking fastidious notes. After eighteen months of studying in French hospitals, she had four professors and the dean of the medical faculty supporting her. Permission to take entrance examinations soon followed.

Dr. Putnam, wearing a smart new dress and a flowered hat, passed both written and oral examinations. For the first time, the École de Médicine enrolled a fully accredited woman student—an American. She graduated with the highest honors in her class.

Feminine history was made in the hallowed halls of the École de Médicine. Two men came to be examined, and two women, Elizabeth Garrett, who had been commuting to Paris, and Mary Putnam. The two young men were judged "passable," a low mark; Elizabeth Garrett, "*bien satisfait*," a high mark; and the American Dr. Putnam, "*trés satisfait*," the highest possible verdict.

Mary Putnam still had her research to complete. A catastrophe brought the work on her thesis to a halt in July 1870, with the outbreak of the Franco-Prussian War. Most foreigners fled from Paris. Though the medical school was closed, Mary stayed on to work as a hospital intern, freeing a male doctor for active duty through the siege of Paris, the bombings, hunger, and incredible hardships. She had fallen in love and was engaged to a French medical student, now a soldier. Her mind dwelt on his hardships. Her mother worried that Mary would marry a French doctor and never come home. By now, Mrs. Putnam, in view of her daughter's sacrifices, wanted Mary to be rewarded with fulfillment of her ambitions as a physician.

The war took its toll, and again Mary decided against marriage. She completed an elegant publishable thesis and at long last received the medical degree.

She returned to New York in 1871 and opened a private practice. Her devoted father proudly drove the nails that fastened the shingle to the window frame of her new office. Dr. Emily Blackwell recruited Putnam to teach therapeutics at the Woman's Medical College of the New York Infirmary.

An invitation to join the New York County Medical Society changed her life. Dr. Putnam set out for a meeting at which new members were to be officially welcomed by the society president, Dr. Abraham Jacobi, professor of children's diseases at New York University.

Mary Putnam was magnetized by this bearded, famous man. Jacobi publicly welcomed Dr. Putnam to the society. She and Jacobi attended future meetings, and he would escort her home on the streetcars. They talked endlessly about their work. Dr. Putnam, awed by Dr. Jacobi's medical knowledge, was especially touched by his biography.

Jacobi, born in Westphalia, Prussia, in 1830, was a sickly child. His mother struggled to save his life and then supported him through the gymnasium and medical studies. In 1848 Jacobi was arrested for revolutionary activity against the German kaiser. Though he was innocent, he spent two years in prison, some of it in solitary confinement. With his best friend, Carl Schurz, he escaped and made his way to New York where he opened his practice. When a patient could pay, he charged $5 for a confinement.

Dr. Jacobi became famous as the father of American pediatrics. He established the first special clinic for children in the country in New York in 1862. Traditionally, doctors treated children with the same medicines and methods as they did adults. One of every twenty-five infants failed to survive the first year of life. Thousands of death certificates of infants gave "teething" as the cause of death. Abraham Jacobi disputed the readiness to attribute all the diseases of infantile life to teething, which he considered a normal life process. Jacobi shocked New York society by chastising those who staged lavish charity balls to support foundling hospitals. He brought statistics revealing that city orphanages were graveyards. In one such loveless environment not a single infant had survived beyond six months of age. He advocated placing children in foster homes. This philosophy spread across America.

Mary Putnam, impressed by Dr. Jacobi's affection for children, asked a friend why Jacobi had never married to have a family of his own. She learned that Jacobi was twice a widower; his first wife died in childbirth, his second wife with her fourth stillborn child.

Dr. Putnam could not conceal her compassion for a man who had buried two wives and five infants. From sympathy her emotions turned to love.

By the time Abraham Jacobi learned of Mary's two previous engagements, he was convinced that the forty-two-year old doctor was the only wife for him. The two doctors were married in 1873 in a City Hall ceremony.

For both doctors, medical writing was a passion. Mary had at times supported herself in Paris by writing stories and novels that had been published in America. When the Public Health Department asked Jacobi to write a book on baby care, Mary turned her editing talents to recording her husband's observations and experiences. Her father's firm, G. P. Putnam, published the book, *Infant Diet*, which generations of mothers came to rely upon with confidence.

Mary founded the Association for the Advancement of Medical Education for Women, continued to lecture on therapeutics at Female Medical College, and had her own growing practice. Delighted to find herself pregnant, she looked forward eagerly to being a mother. The infant was born with defective lungs and died. Dr. Jacobi had lost his sixth child. The couple grieved.

Determined that her husband would have the family he longed for, Mary again became pregnant. The second baby was born in 1875, a blooming child. They named him Ernst. Dr. Jacobi's cup of joy seemed to overflow as the months passed and the child flourished. The loss of the first baby, Mary observed, "makes this one, if possible, all the more precious." Dr. Jacobi's name was familiar in medical circles, but his fame as a doctor gave him no more pleasure than did his family when he had two children, Ernst and Marjorie.

In 1875 Harvard University sponsored an essay contest, the Boylston Medical Prize of $200, for the best paper on "Do women require mental and bodily rest during menstruation?" The topic intrigued Mary Jacobi, who disapproved of the canard that a woman had to lose a week out of every month because she menstruated. She considered it repulsive that a woman could not compete in the professional world because a fourth of her life had to be spent under the influence "of a function in which neither mind nor body are [sic] in a condition to meet professional demands."

Mary had written papers encouraging women to study and observe commonsense rules of good hygiene. Some doctors held that menstruation caused temporary insanity, prohibiting mental activity. Mary pointed out that in hospitals, women doctors and nurses carried on their normal duties and refused to be invalids for a week out of every month. She had seen patients in menstrual misery, but she was far ahead of her time to note the connection between celibacy and physical suffering. In an era when a woman who failed to marry was considered a failure in life, many of them despaired. Mary believed that boredom could actually cause mental breakdowns. And inevitably she concluded that mental and physical activity during menstruation was not only desirable but necessary.

Dr. Putnam Jacobi decided to submit an entry for the prestigious Boylston Medical Prize. Entries would be submitted anonymously, making it impossible for the judges to know if the essay were written by a man or a woman. Using her wide acquaintances among married and single women, rich and poor, she sent out 1,000 questionnaires. Among the questions were "How far can you walk?"

Such answers as "five or six miles easily" and "ten to fifteen if necessary" were common. Mary's paper contained statistics that had previously never been gathered.

When she won the prize, the insulting conclusions of people who had always insisted that women could never contribute to original scientific research received a blow.

Mary Jacobi taught her medical philosophy, so deeply influenced by the French, to the students of the Woman's Medical College of the New York Infirmary. Dr. Emily Blackwell directed the college and proved less good-hearted than her sister, Elizabeth. She was openly critical of Mary's efforts to restructure the curriculum. Mary Jacobi gradually extended the medical studies to four years and established weekly quizzes and extensive laboratory work, as well as services in outpatient medicine and surgery as requirements for graduation.

In 1882 the Post-Graduate Medical School of New York was founded, and Mary Jacobi was appointed to its faculty as lecturer on children's diseases.

By 1883 the Jacobis were known as the first family of American medicine. Their home on 34th Street was a gathering place for young doctors, both men and women. That year, the happiness the couple had shared for ten years ended. Their eight-year-old son died from diphtheria. Abraham Jacobi, one of the nation's leading authorities on diphtheria, was plunged into depression. Mary developed splitting headaches.

The loss of their beloved child had a lasting effect on both doctors. Though Abraham would eventually win acceptance to use the antitoxin that would wipe out diphtheria as a dread disease, he fell into an abyss of grief so inconsolable that sometimes no one could reach him. Mary Jacobi had continued to teach after the tragedy and to mother her daughter and reach out not only to women medical students but also to graduate physicians. Her love for her husband never dimmed, nor her pride in him. She enjoyed reporting an invitation that came to Abraham Jacobi from the German kaiser, offering to forgive Jacobi for escaping from prison if only the good doctor would return to care for the children in the royal nursery. Jacobi hardly mulled the matter over. He promptly wrote back that since New York children needed him as much as the imperial court youngsters, he'd just stay where he was.

Mary Putman Jacobi died in 1906. Abraham Jacobi survived as a widower until 1919. After his death, someone found among his papers the scribbled lines: "If you asked an old man who had been through hard lifelong work and heart-rending scenes, through success, maybe, and endless failures and disappointments, what he craved to be if he began life again, he would, I think, reply, 'Just a modern doctor.' " Mary was of the same mind.

Paula Weideger, a medical author, carried forward Jacobi's research in *Menstruation and Menopause,* published by Knopf in 1967. She examined the physiology and psychology, myths, legends, and reality of two of our last taboos. Even the words tend to be disguised, for women referred to their menses as "the period" or "the curse" or claimed to be "unwell." Once women became professionals, these attitudes changed.

Cicely Williams

At the American Medical Association Convention in 1967, the AMA Council on Foods and Nutrition Award was presented to Dr. Cicely D. Williams for identifying kwashiorkor as one of the most widespread pediatric diseases of the tropics. Dr. Williams, associated with the Oxford Institute for Social Medicine in England, had worked for two decades to adapt Western medical techniques in caring for mothers and children in Africa and Asia.

Cicely was born in 1893. Her father, James Towland Williams, was director of education in Jamaica. Her parents encouraged her and her siblings to value schooling. As a child, she thought she would like to be a nurse, but she was told she did not have the physical stamina for it.

Because of a shortage of doctors during the First World War, forty-one women were admitted to Oxford, Williams among them. She was privileged to study with one of England's great teachers, Sir William Osler. He impressed her with his priorities in medicine. "First, service to the patient. Second, teaching students, medical or nursing. Third, research."

In 1923 Cicely Williams passed her finals at Oxford. She still needed to write a doctoral thesis. She mailed out seventy applications for an internship. The war was over and so was the doctor shortage. No hospital would accept her. Finally she found a place at the South London Hospital for Women and Children, where she assisted with gynecological surgery.

During the two years she was at the South London Hospital, she continued to apply repeatedly for an overseas position. At last she was sent to Africa. She was welcomed with open arms and told that the Colonial Office had been pleading for a decade for a woman doctor, but none had ever applied!

In Koforidua, with no help but one African girl who knew very little English, Dr. Williams attended to over 150 patients, sick children with smallpox, scabies, or severe malnutrition. Mothers brought containers, mostly gin bottles, and Williams taught them to rinse them for the medicine she dispensed. Mothers lined up day after day under the impression that the more often you saw the doctor, the healthier you might become.

The children Cicely Williams examined had swollen legs and bellies, peeling skin, a reddish tinge to the hair, and peculiar rashes. Kwashiorkor, a form of protein malnutrition found in infants and young children, was "the weaning disease," the result of a mother neglecting an older child's diet while nursing a new baby. Other doctors insisted that Dr. Williams was failing to diagnose pellagra. Eventually, Williams would not only identify kwashiorkor but find a cure for it.

"What do you feed the child?" She learned to ask this question in many African languages. A consuming interest in nutrition led her to study kwashiorkor. In areas where animal protein may be difficult to provide in a child's diet, Dr. Williams urged mothers to substitute peanuts, soybeans, and legumes. The improvement in the children's health convinced her she had made an important discovery.

In her African clinic, she examined a dying child with hemolytic streptococcus. When the child passed away, Dr. Williams did a postmortem and accidentally scratched her finger. The next day she was in pain and delirious with fever. She told her colleague she thought she had picked up hemolytic streptococcus, and he belittled the idea. "You'd be dead." But when he aspirated some pus and sent it for culture, he discovered her diagnosis was correct and ordered her immediately to the operating table.

She lay close to death for a long time. When she at last recovered, a superior officer with whom she argued had her shipped off to Kumasi. Cicely Williams had hoped to build a children's unit in the Princess Marie Louise Hospital in Accra, Ghana. Now, disappointed and depressed, she determined to make her year in Kumasi count. She would concentrate on her doctoral thesis for Oxford. Dr. Williams learned that African witch doctors had cures for tetanus and meningitis still unknown in Europe. She observed the devotion of African mothers to their children and was impressed with their powers of lactation. When an infant's mother died, a grandmother who had not had a baby for nineteen years was able to breastfeed the granddaughter.

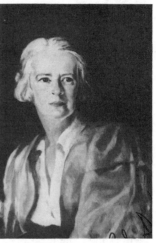

Cicely Williams identified kwashiorkor as one of the most widespread pediatric diseases of the tropics. *(Photo courtesy of Cicely Williams.)*

By the end of the year, Dr. Williams had completed her thesis, "Child Health in the Gold Coast." When Oxford accepted it, she returned to England to receive her medical degree. Proud at last to wear the crimson gown with scarlet sleeves, she believed her father's dream for her was realized; her only grief was that he had not lived to see it.

Cicely's greatest test of courage came when she was transferred by the Colonial Office to Malaya. She had hoped to have a career in Africa; she believed a woman doctor would have little chance for promotion in Malaya.

Then came the war, and bombs fell on Singapore. Williams frantically carried hundreds of sick children from one destroyed building to another. Japanese secret police arrested her and took her to Kempaitai, the Japanese torture headquarters. They repeatedly questioned her, took her glasses, and threatened to torture her. She was the only woman to lecture in the men's prisoner-of-war camp. The Japanese forced her to crawl through a padlocked door two feet high into a cage with seven men and a toilet. The lavatory was the only source of water for washing or drinking. Williams vomited for hours. The prisoners were forced to sit along a bug-infested wall, cross-legged, forbidden even to lean back. One of her longtime friends was in the cell. He had been so badly beaten, his back looked like raw liver. The men cheered her with their support and respect and hid their eyes when she used the toilet. On her birthday, a friend slipped her a sliver of soap—something so precious, she remembered it all her life.

When the long war was over, her ordeal left her so weak she could not walk onto the ship taking her back to England. However, after a long rest in the lovely English countryside, she recovered. She insisted on returning to Malaya to take charge of maternity and child welfare, the highest Colonial Service position ever held by a woman.

Cicely Williams felt a strong bond with young people who expressed distaste for "being corralled into institutions, wards, outpatients, laboratories. They want to see how and where and why and when problems arise. And of course, they are perfectly right. The training of doctors, nurses, and midwives is too much institutionalized. Ornithologists have long recognized that you cannot study birds by studying birds in cages.

"With the domination of institutions has come the preponderance of 'specialists' and 'research.' But to my mind, it's the general practitioner who is badly needed in medicine and in nursing—people who will look after people, not just look after disease.

"Medical care, health services are not just methods of preventing and curing diseases. They are methods of improving the progress of a community. They are peculiarly suitable for women as the study is useful whether or not these women have families of their own." Even if the work proves distressing, Williams said, "It is infinitely worthwhile. Here is a field of work that desperately needs more recruits and more ideas."

Dr. Williams observed that doctors began specializing in pediatrics and created child-welfare centers only in recent decades and only after the major epidemic diseases such as smallpox and cholera were under control. She deplored the fact that in developing countries major epidemic diseases still take their toll.

Dr. Williams, convinced that programs that care for mothers and infants should protect the most vulnerable members of the population, quoted Sir James Spence: "Look after 100 babies and you look after 100 families."

In parts of Africa, she observed, "you cannot get children into the hospital unless you take in mothers as well. You cannot interest people in advice on 'prevention' unless they have confidence in you. When children are dying of malnutrition and gastroenteritis, it is useless to give lectures on boiling the water or opening the windows.

"In the past, medical programs have demanded acquiescence. People remained inactive while rubbish was collected or a house sprayed for mosquitoes. They go to the hospital and passively permit themselves to be vaccinated for a disease, or injected for another, or operated on for a third. These evolutions often remain incomprehensible and mysterious. In this way, people may become submissive to authorities and irresponsible. In parts of West Africa, I know that the sanitary inspector was always known as the 'Summons-Summons man.'"

In her old age, Dr. Williams worried about an African population that was increasing faster than the food supply. She had hoped to live to see the passing of the old tradition of women having twelve children in order to raise six. She had witnessed rural women living in a state of perpetual fatigue.

An African mother may consider her large family indicative of her status and hopes for security when she is elderly. Tribal rivalries are strong. The importance of the tribe depends on its size.

In many African countries, farming remains women's work. The women produce, without oxen, tractors, or even plows, more than 70 percent of the continent's food, according to the World Bank. Men consider the backbreaking hand cultivation "women's work." Men may have two or three wives, all of whom have children. Often the man moves to a town to earn money, there taking on two or three other wives who each have half a dozen children. Wives in a polygamous marriage may be hostile toward each other, but they have to work together anyway. They may have to collect water from some distance, carrying six-gallon cans home on their heads. A baby is carried on the back while the woman digs for food in the hot sun or seeks fast-disappearing wood. Other pervasive inequalities are wife-beating, which is looked upon as normal (how else would she know he loves her?) and sending boys to school while girls remain uneducated.

Jill Seaman

Civil wars wiped out huge populations in Africa in the last decade of the twentieth century. In Sudan's western Upper Nile region, Duar was ravished by Kala-azar (visceral Leishmaniasis), a deadly disease caused by a parasite protozoan. Transmitted by the bite of a sand fly about an inch long, the disease invades and weakens the immune system, causing fever, weight loss, anemia, and enlargement of the spleen. A painful death follows.

Only the heroic intervention of Dr. Jill Seaman, a remarkable American woman from Moscow, Idaho, prevented the epidemic of Kala-azar from becoming a contemporary black death like the plague which ravaged Europe in the Middle Ages. Dr. Seaman had provided health services to Yupik people in Alaska. She was studying at the London School of Hygiene and Tropical Medicine when she was recruited to work in Duar. Working for a Dutch branch of "Doctors Without Borders," she traveled to the most remote areas of the world, governed by the Islamic fundamentalists. War and famines weakened the population. The government banned relief operations, expecting that the disease would prove more effective than armed troops in quelling rebellions.

The trip to Sudan was a nightmare, and when she finally arrived there, she was aghast at what she had signed up for. "My legs," she said, "swelled up to twice their size with mosquito bites." She was stunned by the human disaster. Seaman and Nuer (local) staff members set up operations in Ler. For several days, walking to the village, Seaman and Dutch staff members found dead and dying everywhere. The surviving population were walking skeletons with sick children carrying starving infants.

Seaman spent six months using fans to suck insects into traps to dissect and analyze them. Twice, government forces bombed the Ler vicinity. In November 1991, rebel troops moved through Duar. With 1,400 patients in Duar and 600 more in Ler, the Dutch medical team decided to evacuate.

Some time later, when Seaman returned to Africa, she witnessed a crazed patient throwing a spear into another man's chest. Seaman operated and saved the victim's life. By late 1995, Seaman and the Dutch staff had treated about 19,000 patients, and the epidemic in southwestern Sudan began to subside.

The people, the Nuer, loved Dr. Seaman. One of the most respected head chiefs claimed, "We have named many of our daughters Jill. Now we will also name our sons Jill."

There was a time when the last hut in Duar had been abandoned or destroyed. By 2000, the huts were occupied everywhere, and people expected a decent future.

Jill Seaman's best-known achievement was her effort to introduce birth control in some sub-Saharan African nations, including Kenya, once viewed as a demographic catastrophe. Thanks to the affection and esteem with which Kenyan mothers held Seaman, fertility rates plunged dramatically.

World Fertility Rates

By 2000, fertility rates had plunged in Tunisia, where Muslim women reduced family size from an average 7.2 to 2.9 children in thirty years. In Iran and Syria, rates remained high, but in Bangladesh, the birthrate fell from 6.2 to 3.4 in one decade. From 1968 to 1998, zero population growth was a goal throughout the world. The prevailing idea was that humans were reproducing ominously and population growth was a cancer leading to a depletion of world resources. In Europe during the 1980s, the birthrate was about 1.4 children per mother. By 1998 demographers were astounded at the reduction of fertility in such a nation as Italy, a Catholic country with a fertility rate of 1.2 children per mother. Japanese and Russian rates were 1.4 children per mother.

AIDS in Africa

In Zimbabwe, as in other sub-Saharan African nations, the AIDS problem is so severe it eclipses the overused term "crisis." Not since the horror of the Black Death has there been so great a threat to entire populations, where nearly 40 percent of women coming for HIV counseling test positive. AIDS researchers focused on women rather than men because women have come to trust clinics for care during childbirth and for learning about birth control. In Africa in 2000, research targeted reproductive-age women not yet infected. The goal of the research was to keep women and their families alive.

Originally, more than 10,000 volunteers for the trials were screened for HIV. Additionally, data would be gathered on the incidence of HIV infection in Zimbabwe, a country probably typical of southern Africa.

Zimbabwe's male-dominated culture, struggling with poverty and a lack of medical care, suffers rampant inflation and unemployment. With a history of polygamy, as in other African countries, men go to cities to seek work, leaving behind wives and children. Some wives left behind may sell sex, especially when their children's school fees must be paid. Fathers may pay a son's fee but refuse to pay for their daughters.

An education may sometimes enable a young girl to resist older men with the "three Cs": car, cell phone, and cash. These men believe the girls are less likely than the older women to have HIV, and some even think that having sex with a virgin might cure them of the HIV they have contracted.

"Sexual and hygienic practices in southern Africa also contribute to the high rate of infection," according to Carol Ezzell, writing in *Scientific American* (May 2000). "It is not uncommon for women to use their fingers, cloth, paper, or cotton wool to swab the vaginal walls immediately before and during intercourse to achieve so-called dry sex, which is favored by many men. Some women insert detergents, herbs, and rarely, soil on which a baboon has urinated obtained from traditional healers to induce an inflammatory reaction that dries, warms, and tightens the vagina."

The February 2000 issue of the *Journal of Infectious Diseases* reported that women who use such intravaginal practices were more likely than nonusers to disrupt the normal balance of healthy bacteria in their vaginas. Such disruptions make the vagina more susceptible to sexually transmitted infections.

Another survey of HIV-positive women in Zimbabwe claimed that 67 percent of the women said they experienced pain during sex, and half of those had a sexually transmitted disease or pelvic inflammatory disease.

One aim of the researchers was to get women to use diaphragms that would at least protect against chlamydia and gonorrhea.

In 2000 President Bill Clinton and his administration formally designated AIDS as a threat to governments that might touch off ethnic wars and destroy free-market democracies abroad. The National Security Council would develop a series of expanded initiatives to drive international efforts to combat the disease. African-American leaders, furious at medicines priced beyond the reach of the developing world, were responsible for the new resources.

Susannah O'Reilly

In Sydney, Australia, Susannah Hennessy O'Reilly, the oldest offspring of a physician, was educated at Methodist Ladies' College and the University of Sydney, receiving her M.B. and M.Ch. in 1905. She applied for residency at Sydney Hospital. Although better qualified than many of the men applicants, she was informed there was simply no place to house her. Annually, six doctors completed residency, and their places would be filled by incoming students who had passed examinations in the university medical school.

In 1905 the directors had selected five male students and were considering O'Reilly. The directors agreed that she had a "splendid record." Would appointing a woman be in the best interests of Sydney Hospital? Dr. O'Reilly would be an officer and perhaps would be uncomfortable in the nurses' quarters. Her presence might dampen the spirits of the nurses because her orders had to be obeyed. A member of the board observed that nurses often resented women physicians.

Dr. O'Reilly could be housed in a room outside the hospital, but residents had always conformed to strict discipline and had never been allowed outside hospital premises without permission. Since each resident was assigned special cases, if a patient were suddenly taken ill during the night, it might be difficult to get a woman doctor to the bedside promptly. Would a woman have a restraining influence on her male colleagues? The sixth residency was given to a less qualified man.

A Sydney Hospital volunteer wrote indignantly to the newspaper that she would no longer collect money for the hospital's charities. "It seems we get all work and no money, we women."

Amateur poets flooded the letters-to-the-editor columns of Sydney newspapers:

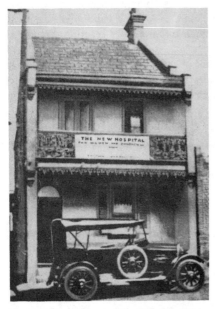

'Tis in the Sydney hospital
which people speak of highly
The doctors hate the doctor gal
Whose name is Sue O'Reilly!
They know she is a gifted aide
And truly skillful in the trade,
But sooth to say,
They seem afraid
Of Doctor Sue O'Reilly!

Undaunted, Dr. O'Reilly accepted an internship at the Royal Adelaide Hospital and later at the Queen Victoria Hospital in Melbourne. Eventually, she joined the staff of the Royal Hospital for Women in Sydney. In 1908 she practiced with her father, and after his death she took charge of his patients.

Having walked into a brick wall of prejudice against women in medicine, O'Reilly enthusiastically supported the founding of the New Hospital for Women and Children in Sydney in 1921.

The first Rachel Forster Hospital, founded by Dr. Lucy Gullett and her colleagues in 1921. (*Photo courtesy of M. Scott Young.*)

That year, Dr. Lucy Gullett attended the twenty-fifth anniversary jubilee celebrations of the Queen Victoria Hospital, which had been established in 1896 by medical women for the care of women and children. Queen Victoria Hospital provided training and practice for women graduates of medical schools who had been unable to get internships. Gullett graduated from the University of Sydney Medical School and had been a resident medical officer at the Children's Hospital in Brisbane. She promoted a similar hospital for Sydney.

During World War I, Gullett drove an ambulance in France and served with a French hospital at Lyons. In 1918, returning with the Australian forces that had fought at the front, she took up practice in Kirribilli. She was appointed honorary physician at the Renwick Hospital for Infants.

Dr. Gullett combined forces with Dr. O'Reilly, Dr. Harriet Biffin, and other Australian women physicians to raise 1,000 pounds to buy a house in a Sydney slum. The doctors themselves scrubbed floors, painted walls, and took up hammers to do the repairs. The hospital opened in 1921; the doctors assumed all responsibilities for administration. The building was so unstable that an overweight patient, for her own protection, was forbidden to leave the ground floor. The hospital served only outpatients and had no beds. The physicians made house calls for seriously ill patients. Their greatest accomplishment was the establishment of a venereal disease clinic, which was still functioning as the largest and most proficient in Australia during World War II.

In 1925 the hospital outgrew its rickety shack and moved to more spacious, better-equipped premises in George Street, Redfern. The name was changed to the Rachel Forster Hospital for Women and Children, honoring the wife of the governor-general who had enjoyed great popularity during his term of office (1920–1925). The Forsters had had four children. Two daughters were married. The family was devastated by the loss of the two sons killed in the war. Since there would be no way of carrying on the name, the women doctors wished to show appreciation for Lady Forster's strong support.

The hospital established well-baby clinics. Eventually men as well as women and children patients were treated by both men and women doctors. Dr. Margery Scott Young taught surgery to male and female residents and, as superintendent of the hospital in the 1970s, saw over 50,000 patients pass through the institution annually.

As in America and England, Australian women doctors deeply influenced the awareness of the kind of health care that ought to be available to everyone.

Canadian Pioneers

Elizabeth Smith

In 1980 the University of Toronto Press published *The Diaries of Elizabeth Smith, 1872–1884*, edited with an introduction by Veronica Strong-Boag. Elizabeth Smith was born in 1859 in Winona, Ontario. Her mother, Isabella McGee Smith, a widowed teacher, had left Nova Scotia hoping to remarry. Elizabeth started her career as a teacher. Influenced by her mother's support of feminist causes, she audaciously decided to leave teaching and study medicine.

At the time, male doctors, in an overcrowded profession, had trouble making a living. The medical men urged women of "modest femininity" to become noble nurses. The few women who insisted on a medical education were advised to devote themselves exclusively to impoverished patients. In 1890 a doctor recorded in the *Canada Medical Record* that poor working women would pay female physicians $4 for confinement and care, while a young medical man had been taught not to deliver an infant at such a low fee. The same professor had taught that a woman doctor "out of the tenderness of her heart could do limitless good by caring for the underprivileged."

Though no woman had graduated with a Canadian medical degree, when Smith applied to the Medical School at Queen's University, she was told she could attend lectures there, but she would not be enrolled. The *Toronto Mail* published a small article suggesting that female students might be accepted at the College of Physicians and Surgeons in Toronto in spring 1878. Elizabeth hurried to take entrance exams. She was devastated at her failure.

Uniform academic standards at the medical schools helped to discriminate against women. In school, girls rarely studied Latin. Another hurdle to acceptance was the increased tuition at better universities. Families expected to provide financial support for a son but few would support a daughter.

Smith considered applying to the medical school in Ann Arbor, Michigan. Drs. Jennie Kidd Trout and Emily Howard Stowe, two early Canadian exponents of women's right to medical training, having been rejected by Canadian medical schools, studied in the United States. Dr. Stowe graduated from the New York Medical College for Women in 1867. Dr. Trout finished eight years later at the Woman's Medical College of Pennsylvania. On returning to Canada, the women physicians had a cold reception from their male colleagues. Aroused, younger women were recruited to reform both the profession and the treatment of patients.

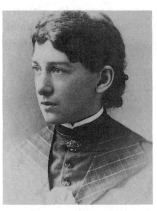

Elizabeth Smith became Dr. Stowe's special disciple. In 1879 Smith again took medical school entrance exams, this time successfully. Hoping to have some female companions in the medical school, she ran an ad in Toronto newspapers asking women interested in medicine to get in touch with her. Among many responses was one from Emily Stowe's daughter, Augusta, who was accepted that fall at the medical school of Victoria University. Augusta, the only woman in the medical program, faced discrimination from day one to the hour of her graduation in 1883.

Three other women, Alice McGillivray, Elizabeth Beatty, and Annie Dickson, joined the incoming class. Close female friendships and strong emotional ties among these women supported them through surgery, medical examinations, and open hostility from male students. The medical school provided separate special classes in obstetrics, anatomy, dissecting, and physiology.

Elizabeth Smith encouraged women to take up medicine as a career. *(Photo courtesy of U. of Toronto Press.)*

In Toronto Dr. Trout and Dr. Stowe promoted the idea of a women's medical school, asking that women be on the board. From her own salary, Dr. Trout guaranteed financial support for such a school on the condition that women share the management and faculty teaching. In 1883 the Kingston Woman's Medical College opened.

Toronto women, not to be outdone by Kingston, launched a fund-raising campaign. The Toronto Woman's Medical College also began admitting students in 1883.

Of the two Canadian establishments, the Kingston institution, where Elizabeth Smith had studied, was much the weaker. Eventually the Toronto school, with finer facilities and greater support, brought about the demise of Queen's school in 1893. Before Queen's closed, Elizabeth Smith, Elizabeth Beatty, and Alice McGillivray graduated in its first class, in 1884. Annie Dickson had left school for a while and graduated in 1886. Dr. Beatty went to India as a Presbyterian medical missionary; Alice McGillivray, class valedictorian, taught anatomy at Queen's; and Elizabeth Smith applied to teach at Toronto, but Augusta Stowe won the position.

Elizabeth started private practice in Hamilton. During the ordeals of her medical studies, she had been supported by a warm friendship with Adam Shortt. The relationship grew into mutual admiration and love.

When Elizabeth received an appointment to lecture in medical jurisprudence at Kingston Woman's Medical College, Shortt promptly accepted a position teaching philosophy at Queen's. They were married at Christmas 1886. When Queen's closed in 1908, Adam had to move his family to Ottawa. Elizabeth devoted herself to rearing her children and to volunteer work, championing the fight against tuberculosis. In Elizabeth's diary, we meet a brave nonconformist full of fun, vivacity, and wit.

Marion Hilliard

Of women physicians honored in Canada, few were more beloved and honored than Marion Hilliard. Born in 1902 in Morrisburg, Ontario, she was educated at the University of Toronto. As chief of Women's College Hospital for ten years and on the hospital staff from 1927 to 1957, she realized her dream of seeing the Woman's College as a teaching hospital, not only for her own department of obstetrics and gynecology, but for every department.

Author of an international best-seller, *A Woman Doctor Looks at Life and Love,* published by Doubleday, Toronto, in 1957, Dr. Hilliard donated all the Canadian royalties to a Women's College Hospital Trust Fund. The book was serialized in magazines and condensations and translated into many languages, including Japanese.

Her colleagues admired her great courage. When she died in 1958, one said, "Dr. Hilliard's practice of medicine was more than a science; it was a great art. Each patient felt that she was the only one who mattered."

Dr. Hilliard was shocked to see how women were treated in childbirth and determined that she would deal with mothers in a humane and sensitive way. In a career in which she delivered as many as fifty babies a month and held forty appointments a day, she earned the love of her patients and found time to do surgery, to write (and beautifully), to give lectures, and to speak on radio. She believed in frank sex education and promoted prenatal clinics. In 1956 in tribute to her, some 1,300 grateful patients subscribed $7,500 toward establishing a medical scholarship fund at her hospital in her name.

Other Canadian Achievers

In the *Nova Scotia Medical Bulletin* (July and August 1955), Muriel G. Currie traced the careers of 14 Canadian women physicians, all born in the late 1800s. Among them, Dr. Margaret Ellen Douglas practiced in Winnipeg and served overseas during the World War I. Dr. Annie Isabel Hamilton practiced in Halifax and later in China. Dr. Maude Elizabeth Seymour Abbott had a distinguished career in cardiology.

In 1974 Carlotta Hacker published *The Indominable Lady Doctors*, marking the golden jubilee of the Federation of Medical Women of Canada. Even as late as 1993, while some Canadian women physicians achieved equality with men in prestige, income, and service, many still faced discrimination. A survey of women doctors revealed that 75 percent of those responding had been sexually harassed by their patients. The doctors were offended by suggestive looks or sexual remarks, by patients touching or brushing against them, or even their inappropriate gifts such as tapes of love songs, G-strings, or the clothes of a dead wife. Though patients' alcohol or drug use may have played a role in sexual harassment, doctors reported that such behavior was "widespread and troublesome."

The survey, conducted by Dr. Susan P. Phillips of Queen's University and psychologist Margaret S. Schneider of the Ontario Institute for Studies in Education in Toronto, involved questionnaires sent to 599 of the 1,064 female family practitioners in Ontario. Replies were received from 417 doctors, 39 percent of the total in the province. The results were published in the *New England Journal of Medicine* in December 1993.

"Female doctors are treated primarily as women, not as physicians, by many male patients," they concluded. "The vulnerability inherent in their sex seems in many cases to override their power as doctors, leaving female physicians open to sexual harassment."

Susan M. Anderson

By 1952 more than half the population of the small town of Fraser, Colorado, had been ushered into the world in the hands of "Doc Susie" who, at eighty-two, was still ministering to the sick and wounded. A tiny, kind, gray-haired woman, she called Fraser home for forty years. It was a town to which she had come to die.

Susan Anderson, born in Indiana in 1870, graduated from the University of Michigan School of Medicine in 1897. She went to Colorado to set up practice because her father was mining in Cripple Creek. He considered Cripple Creek too rough a place for an educated, cultured lady, and after only three years, he convinced her to relocate to Denver. There she eventually set up a practice, working sometimes twenty-two hours at a stretch. Exhausted and sick, she realized she had to rest. She decided to go to Fraser for a brief vacation.

Years later she recalled how she loved Fraser and the double rainbows after soft rains. She returned to Denver reluctantly and again worked to the point of collapse. With self-diagnosis, she was convinced she had tuberculosis. She would return to Fraser; it was as good a place as any to die.

"My first patient in Fraser was a horse who cut himself on a wire fence, and I stitched him up. Those stitches never lasted. The critter tore them out with his teeth. I never got his name, but I pulled him through."

Fraser had only twelve homes and "those generally above a saloon," she recalled. At first, Doc Susie boarded for a while with a storekeeper and then moved into a cabin about the size of a boxcar. However, the community soon learned of her desire to have a log house with a real fireplace. Someone offered her a log building four miles from Fraser if she would have it moved. Doc Anderson went out to inspect it and liked what she saw. She returned with a hammer and a bucket of nails. She drove an eight-penny nail into a log, leaving only the head showing; two nails in the second log, three in the third log, and so on to several hundred. Hammering away, she realized that her health and strength had returned, and she wasn't ready to die yet.

The logs were moved to her lot, and the builder easily put each log in its original place. Doc, using old cardboard boxes, insulated the walls. With great ingenuity she cut glass from a wrecked car for windows. Her patients, friends, and neighbors constructed a beautiful stone fireplace for her.

One Sunday evening some Swedish men arrived with a sled and took her to the Stockholm logging camp to treat a man with a badly cut lip. Doc Susie stitched him up. The Swedish crowd gathered around her, insisting she stay for the dancing. Thoroughly enjoying herself and the music, she wondered about a familiar waltz the fiddlers were playing. "It dawned on me that I had heard that tune when I had seen four horses abreast—*Chopin's Funeral March!*" A drunken Swedish fiddler said he had learned the tune "in the old country." When she explained what it was, the fiddlers were not amused.

Doc Susie, on call day and night, always carried a loaded six-shooter. She walked bravely home from logging camps in pitch-dark or in friendly moonlight. She slept with the six-shooter under her pillow.

One adventurous night, she doctored a sick man who needed to get to his locomotive. Near the rails, she gave a detailed demonstration to the crew manning the train on the proper method of making a stretcher and lifting an injured man. Within the hour, Doc Susie broke several ribs in rescuing her dog, who had crawled into a pit under the train. The very men who had heard her lecture now lifted her properly onto a stretcher.

Another night, a messenger with a sled appeared at her door. A woman in labor needed a doctor in Parshall, twenty-six miles away through canyons and meadows. Doc Susie stretched out on the sled under a blanket. She was taken by sled to catch the train that would take her to a station within a mile of Parshall, a town with no doctor. In bitter cold, on a road that was half mud and half snow, she was carried by sleigh to Williams Fork, where she delivered the youngest son of the Milner family.

"No doctor likes delivering a baby in a kitchen but usually I had no choice."

She recalled that miners were a bit "bashful about having their bar room wounds sewed up by a lady." She rescued abandoned babies and treated men who may have been robbers and murderers. She taught hygiene to women from distant bawdy houses. She vaccinated whole families, even those who could not pay. She traveled to patients through raging blizzards and dark nights when the thermometer quivered at sixty-five degrees below zero. She hiked up 13,000-foot-high mountains to care for timber workers who had broken an arm or a leg. Without assistance, she delivered babies and performed difficult surgery.

Like many women doctors, she repeatedly had to prove she could offer good medicine. She had pride in the "great school from which I graduated and was determined not to bring shame on it."

In the frigid cold of Fraser, Doc Susie wore what everyone else did: long boots and heavy long thermal underwear. Though admittedly never much of a skier, she certainly used skis. She also used snowshoes, sleighs, horses, and vehicles to get to her patients. Once, when townspeople thought she was lost, they sent search parties out for her. "I wasn't lost," she insisted. Indeed she was not. She knew where she belonged. "I guess I was born to be a doctor." She died in 1982.

Sarah Stockton

Sarah Stockton, born on a farm in Tippecanoe County, Indiana, in 1842, graduated from the Woman's Medical College of Pennsylvania in Philadelphia in 1882. For many years, she was in private practice in Indianapolis, and for a time she was physician in charge at the Indiana Women's Prison. At the turn of the century, she joined the staff of the Indiana Central Hospital for the Insane, where she remained for twenty-five years. For her intelligence, dedication, and native feelings, she had the loving respect of the community. Though she outlived the members of her immediate family, she was mourned at her death by a wide circle of friends in 1924.

7

One University's Contributions:
Those Remarkable Johns Hopkins Women

For those who belong here and those to
come, I exult to be ready for them.
Walt Whitman, *Leaves of Grass*

Dr. Mary Putnam Jacobi and her husband were convinced that women would be admitted to medical schools when those who held philanthropic purses put strings on their endowments. Maybe money would talk where ability and determination were mute. This theory was tested when Johns Hopkins Medical School hit a financial iceberg. A philanthropist, Johns Hopkins, had donated $7 million to be divided between a university and a hospital. The university opened in 1876. Fourteen years later, the medical school was still in the talking stage. Trustees begged for money. Though money soon appeared, the trustees did not like the looks of Santa Claus. They had never seen Ms. Claus!

Mary Garrett

Baltimore, the home of Johns Hopkins University, was the hub of a movement for higher education for women in 1890. An heir to a fortune from the Baltimore and Ohio Railroad, Mary Garrett had helped finance Bryn Mawr School. The curriculum of Bryn Mawr matched that of the undergraduate and graduate departments of Johns Hopkins. Garrett realized that the financial problems of the Johns Hopkins Medical School might be an ill wind that would blow women into the most advanced college in America. The Johns Hopkins trustees, frankly skeptical when they were offered $200,000 for a hospital, questioned how women could raise that much money.

Garrett contributed $10,000 to start the ball rolling and launched a "Women's Fund for the Higher Medical Education of Women." By October

1890, the trustees were offered $100,000 if women were admitted to Johns Hopkins. The southern trustees, absolutely courteous to the women, were also absolutely opposed to coeducation at Johns Hopkins. The fund-raisers, all of them marriageable, but all unmarried, were equally adamant.

Two members of the group, Mamie Gwinn and Elizabeth King, had fathers on the board. Aha! Both fathers supported their daughters. The board agreed that if the women could raise $500,000, the sum needed to open the medical school, women would be admitted. But listen to this: the board hedged insultingly, "We're satisfied that in hospital practice among women, in penal institutions in which women are prisoners, in charitable institutions in which women are cared for, and in private life when women are to be attended, there is a need and place for learned and capable women physicians." In other words, women physicians could practice on women patients where there was little or no income.

In 1892 Mary Garrett donated $307,000, which fulfilled the $500,000 needed to open the medical school. Again she stipulated that medical students had to meet the requirements for admission to the graduate school of Johns Hopkins. They would be required to have passed premedical courses. They had to read, write, and speak French and German. The trustees objected at such stiff terms. Fathers of male applicants almost broke down and wept when they pleaded with Garrett to relax her requirements and conditions for her donation. Such high entrance requirements prompted a faculty member to observe, "We are lucky to get in as professors, for I'm damn sure we could never get in as students."

Garrett insisted that women be admitted on the same terms as men. Men and women were to have a four-year rather than a three-year course leading to the degree of medical doctor. The Johns Hopkins Hospital began serving the public four years before the medical school opened in 1893. Harvard, the University of Michigan, and the University of Pennsylvania already had four-year plans, with an eight-month school year.

About this time, a University of Michigan professor was asked if women could enroll in the medical school. He responded, "No, thank God. They can only enter there in the pickling vat."

At last the Johns Hopkins Medical School opened, coeducational. From its beginning Johns Hopkins women distinguished themselves in scholarship.

Florence Sabin

Among those who entered the fourth class at Johns Hopkins Medical School was Florence Sabin. Her anatomy professor, Dr. Franklin Mall, recognized Sabin's unusual talents. He suggested she investigate the origin of lymphatic vessels. Sabin's discoveries about lymph had an explosive impact on medical science.

Sabin's biography is an affirmation of opportunities and responsibilities in a democracy. She had to struggle for a place in the world. It was no joke that she christened her first car "Susan B. Anthony."

Born in 1871, Florence grew into a fuzzy-haired, awkward child who looked through thick glasses out of the ill-fitting windows of a shaky frame house on a mountain in Silver City, Colorado. When she was five years old, a baby brother was born. He lived only a year, and on Florence's seventh birthday, her mother died a few days after the birth of another baby who survived only a year. Florence and her sister Mary, nine, were sent to boarding schools.

In their motherless childhood, the two sisters moved from Denver to Vermont to Chicago and back to their grandparents' Vermont farm. In these moves, Mary provided the only continuity in Florence's life. By the time she was ready for college, she was regarded as a warm, trusting young woman. Both sisters studied at Smith College, where sharp differences seemed to have developed between them, and intense sibling animosities aroused in Florence a lifelong interest in psychiatry. Later in life, Florence became a mother figure to her older sister, and they exchanged frequent letters unmarred by hostility or bitterness.

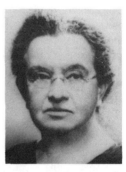

Florence Sabin, the first woman professor at Johns Hopkins University. *(Photo courtesy of Johns Hopkins University.)*

Florence graduated in 1893, convinced she was too homely for any man ever to marry her. She taught school for three years and applied to Johns Hopkins Medical School. By 1900 she was one of two women interns in the hospital, and two years later she was appointed to the faculty. In 1917 she became the first woman professor at Johns Hopkins. Eventually, she headed the histology department, but the road was not always smooth. She had long denied she had been a victim of discrimination, but when a young doctor was promoted over her, she faced the truth that women's achievements were rarely recognized. She devoted herself to encouraging young gifted women. Her efforts on behalf of the women's movement of the 1920s influenced the National Academy of Sciences. In 1921 Madame Marie Curie visited the United States to receive a number of honorary degrees and a gram of radium—a gift funded by a women's magazine. The National Academy of Sciences debated the possibility of electing Madame Curie an honorary member. But Curie, a woman who eventually received two Nobel Prizes, was rejected.

In 1923 medical scientists at the National Academy nominated Florence for membership, but she was not elected. In 1925 the American Association of Anatomists elected her as its first woman president and again nominated her for the National Academy. At last she received this honor. The same year, she became the first woman to be a member of the Rockefeller Institute staff. Dr. Simon Flexner greeted her as "one of the foremost scientists of all time."

Dr. Sabin always helped young scholars at Johns Hopkins Medical School to examine new problems, ideas, and techniques. Generous with her time, she rarely allowed her name to appear on first publications, even as coauthor. Such unselfishness endeared her to her students. When they were well launched in their careers, she often collaborated with them and lent her famous name as coauthor of the published papers of research jointly accomplished.

Sabin's apartment on a hillside in Baltimore reminded her of her Silver City origins. Students found a warm welcome there, and her biographer, Lawrence S.

Kubie, wrote she had her guests helping with meals or sitting on the floor with a stopwatch with orders to turn the steaks at three minutes. In her last years, dignity lent beauty that she had been denied in her youth. Retiring from the Rockefeller Institute in 1938, Florence Sabin returned to the Colorado mountains she loved. There she launched a successful campaign against tuberculosis and other diseases in Colorado. Her legacy in medicine was in three areas: her research into the anatomy of the brain, her research into the embryology of the lymphatic system, and at the end of her life, her efforts to improve the health of the people of Colorado. She died in 1953.

Louise Pearce

Louise Pearce was born in 1885. She graduated from Stanford in 1907, and after earning a Johns Hopkins medical degree in 1912, she joined the staff of Johns Hopkins Hospital. She became a member of the Rockefeller Institute, a position she held until her retirement.

Dr. Pearce led a research team to the Belgian Congo to study sleeping sickness. As a result of her discovery of a drug to conquer the disease, in 1920 she was awarded the Order of the Crown of Belgium. Thirty years later, she was honored with the King Leopold II Prize and the Royal Order of the Lion. Dr. Pearce also made significant contributions in the area of tumor studies and venereal diseases. Many doctors remembered her as the much-loved president of the Woman's College of Pennsylvania. She died in 1959.

Helen Taussig

Best known as the codeveloper (with Dr. Alfred Blalock) of an operation to save the lives of newborns with congenital malformation of the heart (blue babies), Dr. Helen Taussig pioneered in pediatric heart surgery. Taussig, born in 1898, was one of the most honored women physicians in the world. The French made her a Chevalier of the Legion of Honor; Lyndon B. Johnson presented her with the Medal of Freedom, the highest civilian award an American president can bestow. From Athens, Greece, to Oxford, Ohio, twenty colleges presented honorary degrees to Dr. Taussig.

With all this recognition, she claimed that winning awards could not compare to the excitement of donning a sterile cap, mask, and operating gown to observe a surgeon making a "blue baby turn pink."

As a young woman, Taussig faced an almost insurmountable obstacle: being female. "I grew up in an atmosphere that greatly differs from that of today. Fifty years ago, an error made by a woman was held against her, whereas any error made by a man was just a mistake!"

She was born into a family of scholars in Cambridge, Massachusetts, in 1898. Her mother was one of the first graduates of Radcliffe College. Her father, Frank William Taussig, a famous economist at Harvard, acted as an advisor to President Woodrow Wilson.

Taussig enrolled at Radcliffe with little in-terest in having a medical career. She studied biology and physics but majored in tennis. To get away from cold winters in New England, Helen and two friends transferred to the University of California in Berkeley in 1921. When she told her father she wanted to be a doctor, he sug-gested she might do better in public health and urged her to apply to the Harvard School of Public Health, which was to open in the fall of 1922. Harvard Medical School made no bones about opposing the admission of women. When Taussig was interviewed at the School of Public Health, the dean told her women could indeed study there, but they would not be awarded a degree.

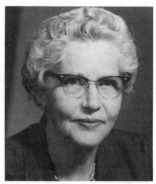

Helen Taussig faced discrimination at Harvard University. *(Photo cour-tesy of The Passano Foundation.)*

Who would be so foolish to spend years studying medicine, knowing all the while she'd never be able to use the knowledge in a profession?

Indignant, the young Taussig enrolled at Harvard to study histology. She was required to sit in a far corner of the room by herself and to refrain from speaking to male students. To examine slides, she was assigned to a separate room with her microscope.

Taussig had to transfer to Boston University to study anatomy. Fortunately, Dr. Alexander Begg recognized great potential in this young woman. One day he thrust the heart of a calf into her hand. "It won't do you any harm to get in-terested in one of the larger organs of the body as you go through medical school," he said.

Greatly encouraged, Taussig dissected the heart. Dr. Begg suggested she ap-ply to Johns Hopkins. Taussig, annoyed that the head of Boston University Medical School would urge a fine student to apply elsewhere, acted on his ad-vice. She was accepted by Johns Hopkins, and when the time came to choose a medical specialty she chose internal medicine. She lost out on that choice to another woman student, but she won a fellowship in the adult cardiac clinic. She began investigating congenital malformation of the heart. In the meantime, she decided she would prefer to be a pediatrician.

By 1930 Taussig had been appointed head of the cardiac clinic of the child-ren's unit at the Harriet Lane Home. Here she launched her studies of rheumatic fever, a disease that causes inflammation of joints and frequent complications of heart damage in children. In that era, the only treatment for rheumatic fever was simply bedrest and aspirin to keep the strain off the heart so it would not enlarge. In 1935 a baby with bluish skin was brought to Dr. Taussig. Examining the child with an electrocardiography machine, Helen thought one of the baby's heart chambers was missing. Later, another baby's X rays revealed a similar malformation.

"Then and there," Dr. Taussig recalled, "I realized that malformations of the heart repeat themselves and that similar malformations cause familiar changes in the size and shape of the heart."

Obsessed by that realization, she worked with Dr. Alfred Blalock at Johns Hopkins. After two years of operating on animals successfully, Dr. Taussig believed the time had come to try the operations on blue babies.

Their third operation was on a "small, utterly miserable, six year old boy" no longer able to walk. When she located the leak in his heart, the anesthesiologist cried, "He's a lovely color now!" Taussig walked around to the head of the operating table and was thrilled to see that the patient had normal pink lips. Within days, the child was healthy, happy, and active.

Taussig and Blalock observed many oxygen-deprived infants and children who might be helped by increased circulation to the lungs. The doctors theorized that a deficiency of oxygen in the bloodstream caused the syndrome, and it could be alleviated by grafting two major arteries together. The surgery changed the cyanotic infant from blue to a "lovely normal peach color." They operated on many congenital malformations of the heart. By demonstrating that even the deeply cyanotic child could survive heart surgery, the two doctors demonstrated that almost any patient might do so. Heart surgeons began to venture where they had previously not dared to go.

In 1945 Blalock and Taussig published the results of their studies of blue baby operations. Dr. Blalock won recognition and election to the National Academy of Sciences. For Dr. Taussig recognition came more slowly. Her first honorary degree in 1948 was from Boston University, where she had held the calf heart in her hand. She became full professor at Johns Hopkins in 1959 and was elected by the American Heart Association as its first female president.

In 1962 a German student, Dr. Aloes Beuren, mentioned that a number of deformed babies had been born in Germany and other European countries. Dr. Taussig, mulling over the conversation, decided to go to Germany to check out the sleeping pill that Dr. Beuren had mentioned as a possible cause of the malformations. In Germany and England, Taussig visited clinics, interviewed doctors, and examined malformed children. Dr. Taussig was soon convinced that these terrible deformities had to be linked to the pill thalidomide. On her return to the United States, she spread the alarm, warning physicians of the danger of thalidomide and similar drugs, probably saving thousands of infants from birth malformations. She died in 1985.

Jennifer Niebyl

Women researchers at Johns Hopkins continued to explore the cause of deformities in infants. In 1979 research revealed that some drugs, vitamin deficiencies, or exposure to environment gases could increase the risk that mothers with cleft-lip children would give birth to another child with a similar defect.

Dr. Jennifer Niebyl, director of the study, canvassed the nation for mothers of children with cleft lips. Mothers planning to have another baby could provide a clue to the cause of the second most common birth defect in the United States.

"We know that there's a strong genetic tendency in the cleft-lip syndrome," claims Dr. Niebyl, "but the risk is 1:20 of cleft lip appearing in a subsequent pregnancy. What we're really looking for is what environmental or metabolic factors could influence the expression of the defect."

Was there something in the environment or in a mother's body that influenced her chances of having another defective child? Dr. Niebyl claimed that paint fumes, hair spray, drugs, and anesthetic gases could cause recurrences of the

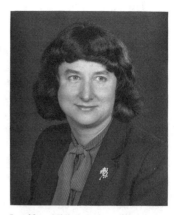

Jennifer Niebyl was director of maternal-fetal medicine at Johns Hopkins. *(Photo courtesy of Jennifer Niebyl.)*

condition. Tests on laboratory mice found that high dosages of vitamin A and a number of chemicals and drugs, including cortisone and dilantin (a drug taken by epileptics), produced offspring with cleft-lip defects.

In 1982 Niebyl became director of maternal-fetal medicine at Johns Hopkins School of Medicine. She coedited a textbook of obstetrics. Her book *Drug Use in Pregnancy* was republished in a second edition. In 1998 she was appointed professor and chair of the Department of Obstetrics and Gynecology. Such research gives continuity to the high purpose for which Johns Hopkins was founded.

Hilde Bruch

During her years as clinical professor of psychiatry at Baylor University Medical College in Houston, Dr. Hilde Bruch was one of the best-known authorities on the psychological aspects of obesity and other eating disorders. Dr. Bruch considered psychiatry a particularly congenial profession for women. "When I was born in 1904 in Germany, anyone who was qualified could get accepted to medical school. A higher percentage of women were accepted. If you ask me if there is prejudice where patients refused to go to women doctors, I am sure some men would never go see a woman physician. I wouldn't have had occasion to meet such men. Before I was a psychiatrist," she reflected smiling, "I was a pediatrician, and I'm sure women pediatricians treat as many boys as girls."

Bruch had been motivated to study medicine because of her curiosity. "I was a teenager when I first learned that girls could go to the university. I decided that was what I wanted to do. I was good in mathematics and wanted to major in math. But an uncle vetoed that idea. He said, 'You'll get only high school teaching or boring jobs with no future. Why not study medicine?'

"Higher mathematics would never have been as stimulating as medicine for me. I like working with people. My uncle said if I tried to go into higher mathematics I would run into prejudice because of my religion rather than because of my sex. What does one know at eighteen? We cannot foresee what it means to live with a profession. I made a good choice; there are so many exciting aspects of medicine from which to choose!

"Shortly after talking to my uncle, I went ice skating. The medical students skimming around on the ice wore their class caps—the fellows wearing red caps, the girls wearing crimson berets. I was envious of those berets! That may have prompted my application to medical school. I wanted the right to wear one of those crimson berets. Anyway, in a few months I was wearing one!"

In Europe universities were more freewheeling than in America. Dr. Bruch thought a student had more freedom to choose subjects, study on her own, and select courses. Of course, students had been through a more rigid, structured, highly disciplined high school and had learned to study. They fulfilled certain minimum requirements. In medical school, a student could take four, five, even six, years to finish the regime. Early upbringing and education had been demanding, and only top students could go to a university.

"Students took lab work and showed up for ward assignments, naturally, but the responsibilities for study, the testing of knowledge, was left up to the medical student. No one shadowed a medical student in Europe. I think women tended to be more conscientious than the men. American women medical students also seem to be more conscientious. In the past, restricted admissions forced the American women to work harder."

Dr. Bruch graduated from the University of Freiburg and completed an internship in Germany. By the advent of the Hitler regime, her family had to flee Germany. "We arrived in America in the midst of the Depression. You cannot imagine the situation. No positions available, and most German-Jewish refugees arrived with valuable professional training and experience." In 1934 Dr. Bruch worked at New York Babies Hospital where there were already three or four women on the staff. Three were Johns Hopkins graduates; they encouraged her to apply to work and study at Johns Hopkins, where she met a matter-of-fact attitude toward women physicians.

In the half century that Dr. Bruch worked as a doctor, she continued to be grateful to her uncle who had steered her toward the profession. "He was absolutely right," she said. "The great joy of my life is being a medical woman." She died in 1984.

Gertrude Stein

Gertrude Stein was encouraged by William James to apply to Johns Hopkins Medical School. Nine years earlier, four Baltimore women had heavily endowed the university on condition that women be admitted on the same terms as men. Though she had never passed Latin, Gertrude was accepted, but she soon found that she detested obstetrics. She delivered a number of black babies and absorbed the rhythms of the speech of black mothers. Later she used the dialect in her stories.

Some of Gertrude Stein's professors gave her good grades because they recognized her intelligence. But others were unimpressed by her sloppy laboratory techniques. She was always stained up to the elbows in whatever dye she used. Gertrude Stein flunked out. A professor encouraged her to take a summer course and pick up her class work in the fall. She needed only one more semester to get her medical degree. But she stubbornly refused. "Gertrude, Gertrude," her friends pleaded, "remember the cause of women!" But Gertrude insisted medical school bored her to death. Dr. Florence Sabin, a fellow student at Johns Hopkins, remembered a model of a brain that Gertrude had constructed. It was so fantastic, the professor pitched it into a waste basket.

A celebrated author and art collector, Stein died in 1946 in Paris.

Claribel Cone

Born in 1864, Claribel Cone graduated at the head of her class in 1890 from Baltimore Woman's Medical College. She won one of five internships at the Philadelphia Hospital for the Insane (a plum in an age when women were barred from hospitals on any excuse). She interned at Blakely Hospital for the Insane in Philadelphia and later studied at the new Johns Hopkins University Medical School. From 1894 to 1903 she pursued research at Johns Hopkins and taught pathology at the Woman's Medical College.

Claribel and her sister Etta, daughters of a wealthy businessman, could afford to travel widely. The sisters gained entry to the art world in Paris through Gertrude Stein and her brother, Leo. Today the Cone collection of Matisses fills five galleries of the

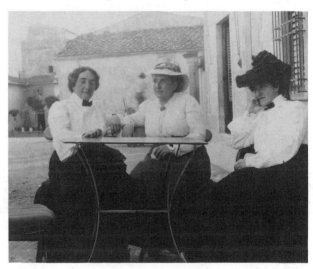

The Cone sisters, with Gertrude Stein (center), became passionate collectors of art. (*Photo courtesy of Baltimore Museum of Art.*)

Cone Wing of the Baltimore Museum of Art, and Dr. Claribel Cone is better remembered as an art collector and personal friend of Gertrude Stein than as a doctor.

Yoshiye Togasaki

The first Japanese woman to graduate from Johns Hopkins Medical School was Yoshiye Togasaki, who was among the Japanese Americans evacuated from the West Coast for internment during World War II. While the rounding up of these U.S. citizens has seared the conscience of the nation since the end of the war, little attention has been paid to the nursing training of many young women among the internees. After the war, some became nurses, and a few went on to medical school.

In *Democracy on Trial: The Japanese Evacuation in World War II,* Page Smith writes about Yoshiye Togasaki, born in San Francisco, the fifth of eight children, who was one of the women inspired to have a medical career. When she was young, she and her sister were sent to Japan to live with their maternal grandmother in Tokyo. Her grandmother was alone, and Togasaki's mother could not cope with the care of eight children while helping her husband run his store.

After the death of her grandmother, Togasaki and her sister returned to the U.S. When she finished high school, she studied at the University of California, Berkeley. Having helped care for sick internees in the camps, she applied to Johns Hopkins Medical School, where she graduated with an unusually fine record.

Stella Robertson

In 1888 the commissioner of patents compiled a list of women inventors to whom patents were issued between 1790, when the first U.S. patent was granted, and 1888. The compilation revealed that during that period, almost 24,000 patents were issued to inventors with feminine names, or approximately 6 percent out of a total of about 400,000. Although some scholars suggest there were many errors of omission in this list, women inventors were a distinct minority. Inventors and researchers in every scientific area were regarded as white males. Today, in medical and engineering courses, women are as likely as not to be at the head of their class and highly visible in important careers.

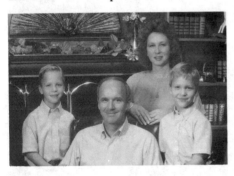

Stella Robertson happily combines a family life and a career. *(Photo courtesy of Stella Robinson.)*

In 1981 Stella Robertson cracked the glass ceiling when she was appointed to the ophthalmic and lens care production department at Alcon Laboratories in Fort Worth, Texas. Over the years, she established the immunology and cell biology units and launched an integrated biotechnology research program, working in monoclonal antibody, biochemistry, and ocular tissue culture programs. She has been in charge of new pharmaceuticals moving from the research lab to commercial sales. She dealt with the U.S. Food and Drug Administration in Washington and with the European Union in Brussels.

"Research," Robertson said, "is like having a pregnancy and then rearing the child. I love it all. Normally, it takes 12 years from the time the drug is discovered to the time it receives approval and gets on the market. My team at Alcon has been lucky in shortening that period. I coordinate projects for pharmaceuticals to treat eye problems and allergies. My group experiments with other drugs as well.

"I was the first person hired at Alcon for these units. In turn, I hired scientists and soon expanded into leading the Allergy and Inflammation research units. Out of this group, we discovered five compounds for which Alcon obtained or filed patents."

In 1993 the Food and Drug Administration approved two of Robertson's R&D team's pharmaceutical creations, Iopidine 0.5% and Alomide, for treating advanced glaucoma and severe allergy. In 1994 Stella and coworkers patented a monoclonal antibody to *Haemophilus* influenza–Type B, prepared from lymphoid and myolema cells. That same year, a second patent was issued for immunoassay of antigens involved in ophthalmic disorders such as *Herpes simplex* virus, adenovirus, chlamydia, and even fungi. Later research contributed to pharmaceuticals designed to prevent corneal scar formation. Stella points with pride to her group's landmark study of a novel immunomodulating drug, Leflunomide, for treating illeitis.

A tall, fair-skinned woman with a calm manner, Stella brings the warmth of an interest in others and a pleasant temperament to serve the demands of her research. Robertson graduated from Goucher in Towson, Maryland, in 1971 cum laude with a double major in biology and education. She received a Ph.D. in molecular biology and immunology from Johns Hopkins in 1978. Always interested in science, Stella had a difficult decision to make: would she have a profession in medicine or science?

"As my research group grew larger," she said, "though the project was developed and conceived in my lab, we would rotate authorship so others would get credit. Most science today is done as a team in academics. My goal is definitely in industry, and as a good science major, I make it a point to be sure others receive due credit."

By 1994 Dr. Robertson had published innumerable abstracts for journals and more than seventeen papers in *Current Eye Research, Lancet, Gastroenterology, Investigative Ophthalmology, Visual Science,* and *Agents and Actions,* among others. She had also contributed to nine books.

Stella embraces two lives—one as scientist, the other as wife and mother. She and Jamie Robertson, also intensely career-minded, met while Stella was at Johns Hopkins. They decided to postpone marriage until he finished his degree. After the wedding, they agreed that Stella would complete her graduate degree, a decision that pleased both his parents and hers. Jamie accepted work for ARCO, a Texas petroleum company, while Stella continued her graduate work in Baltimore. For two years they made that long-distance commute.

"I think of our marriage as traditional," Stella smiles, "though we are definitely a two-career family. We both hold jobs that are time-consuming and demanding."

Her husband's position carried heavy responsibilities, and he was strongly
involved in the Society of Exploration Geophysicists (SEG). Jamie was inaugu-
rated in Los Angeles in 1994 as the SEG's president, and Stella had an important role as they toured the world in 1995. She accompanied him on most of his
business trips such as one to China, where they took time off together to hike in
the rain on the Great Wall.

Stella and Jamie Robertson were thrilled when they had sons, identical
twins, after many disappointing and sobering difficulties with her pregnancies.

Stella averred, "I'd have been happy to have had a daughter, because the
women have been so strong in our family. They have made real contributions to
society. My grandmother was born after the Civil War, went to college, and
taught elementary school until she married in 1902. She started one of the first
Girl Scout troops in Mississippi and raised six children on her own after she was
widowed during the Depression.

"My mother graduated from the University of Mississippi in 1929 with a
B.A. and an M.A. in English and was the first woman selected for the University
Hall of Fame. She went on to Tulane and earned an M.S. in Social Work. Back
in Mississippi, she drove for 13 years around back country roads in Model Ts,
supervising the first Child Welfare Services programs in the state. She married
and had two children after the age of 40. She returned to social work at the
HEW (Department of Health, Education and Welfare) in Washington, D.C. At
85 she had a third career as grandmother to my twins.

"My father," Stella said, "was first a chemist and naturalist, and finally, professionally, a political scientist, an attorney, and a real estate broker in Washington. A champion chess player and an Eagle Scout, he was committed to the philosophy of Boy Scouts.

"Later in life, he also taught real estate courses. From the time I was 8, I
helped him assemble papers. At 15, I got my own real estate license. He influenced my respect for good business practices. 'Know thyself,' he always said.
He always encouraged me to be all I could be.

"My husband was the only male in his generation. Both his parents were
practicing physicians in OB-GYN until they turned 70. They remain active in
Planned Parenthood. At 78 his widowed mother, Ruth, was still working part-
time as an M.D. at the Westchester Hospital. She trained at the University of
Michigan, 1939, one of only eight women in her medical school class."

Robertson's earliest degrees were in biology and education. She was a postdoctoral research fellow of the Arthritis Foundation in the Department of Microbiology, University of Texas Health Science Center at Dallas (UTHSCD).
Since joining Alcon, Stella maintains a relationship with UTHSCD as an adjunct
assistant professor in the Department of Ophthalmology.

In 1993, with her sons in the second grade, she and Jamie were normal
parents attending school plays and helping the boys work on computers. The

Robertsons took the boys on their first ski trip. By their second year at ski school, the twins navigated down the mountain at Keystone, Colorado, like pros.

Stella's life is an illustration of a modern woman combining an exacting profession with being a successful wife and mother.

Stella Robertson and I met on a tour of Paris, and it was instant friendship. This chapter is based on an interview at the 1994 Society of Exploration Geophysicists conference in Los Angeles.

Virginia Apgar

Virginia Apgar, the first woman physician to hold a full professorship at Columbia University, where she taught anesthesiology, also pursued research as clinical professor of pediatrics at Cornell and as a fellow at Johns Hopkins University.

Apgar is best remembered for conducting experiments that led to the development of a simple test. Taken at one minute and at five minutes after a baby's birth, the test predicts an infant's chances for healthy survival. This "Apgar Score" sought to understand factors underlying birth defects and pregnancy failures. Because periodic blood samples were taken from the women involved in Dr. Apgar's impressive projects, it became possible to check for ten known viruses during pregnancy. One infection at least, that of German measles, was well-known as endangering an unborn child. Most children develop immunity to German measles. However, Dr. Apgar's studies revealed that 15 percent of the pregnant women had never had the disease. Exposure to German measles causes serious abnormalities in as many as 40 percent of exposed fetuses. Protection for the fetus against measles can be had by injecting the mother, but doctors worried that the rubella vaccine would harm the fetus itself.

The successful development of the rubella vaccination against German measles is an example of the values and justification for such research. Nevertheless, there are always people who view mass vaccination as contributing to the increased incidence of diabetes and other chronic diseases and disabilities. Fewer than 10 percent of doctors report serious health problems following vaccination of their patients.

Measles, now rare in America, continues to be a threat elsewhere around the world, mostly in developing nations. The disease affected some 30 million children in 2001. For some it is deadly.

In 1982 parents of vaccine-injured children founded the National Vaccine Information Center, hoping to prevent vaccine injuries and deaths through public education and safety reforms. Concern that the rise in autism may have affected one in 500 children has turned the spotlight on a theory that the MMR (measles-mumps-rubella) vaccine may trigger the problem. In 2000 studies focused on the question: why did some children develop autism while others handled the MMR vaccination well? Most parents accept the doctor's assurance that vaccines are safe and life preserving and should remain part of public health policy.

With some 500,000 new cases every year, leprosy continues to be a chronic bacterial infection in India, Asia, Africa, and South America. For these challenging problems there are no easy answers.

Throughout the world, maternal neonatal tetanus, a bacterial infection causing muscle seizures, may be responsible for 215,000 deaths annually. The bacteria exist in soil and probably will never be wiped out. However, vaccinating women of childbearing age may help prevent the spread of the disease.

Polio, after decades of seriously crippling people of all ages, was practically eliminated in the developed countries, thanks to an inexpensive vaccine. In 1988 in India, 1.3 million children were vaccinated in a single day at a cost of twenty cents per patient. By the twenty-first century, the virus had not been completely eliminated, but it shows signs of becoming as rare as smallpox.

8

Oh, Brave New World:
Nobel Prize Winners in Medicine

Oh, brave new world
That has such creatures in it!
Shakespeare, *The Tempest*, Act V, Scene I

Marie Curie

"The image of Madame Curie is overdone," snapped Valentine Telegdi of the University of Chicago. "If I'd have been married to Pierre Curie, I would have been Madame Curie too."

What arrogance! Only a man would make such an observation, retorted a member of the panel of the American Physical Society. "Pierre was a genius, but Madame Curie's persistence led her to a brilliant discovery of radium. On her own! Pierre Curie joined his wife's research, not the other way around. After her husband died, Marie Curie carried on the work and won a second Nobel Prize five years later!"

Gloria Lubkin, a nuclear physicist and then senior editor of *Physics Today* observed, "When I was a youngster, I was inspired by Marie Curie."

Two of the greatest medical discoveries of the nineteenth century were made by women, neither of whom was a doctor.

Marie Curie and Lise Meitner were both physicists and among the most gifted scientists of all time. Madame Curie's discovery of radium, like Lisa Meitner's of nuclear fission, came in a form that only incidentally had medical applications. But the work of these women changed the whole picture of modern science.

Manya Sklodovska was born in Poland in 1867. She went to France to study and combine a scientific career with a flourishing family life. We have to note that in France, the Napoleonic Code had long bound a woman in a cell of obedience to her husband. Article 1124 said the "unfit persons according to law are minors, ex-convicts, and married women." Article 1428 gave the husband the right to administer his wife's money.

Women were legally children. A woman could not even give permission to a doctor to operate on her child without the father's consent. It was not until 1910 that French women were allowed to take the baccalaureate examinations, a prerequisite to university entrance.

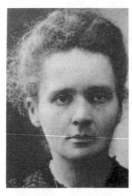

Young Manya Sklodovska (Marie Curie) dreamed of studying medicine in Paris. *(Photo courtesy of Institute Curie, Paris.)*

Curie was born Manya Sklodovska, the daughter of a Warsaw science teacher. She had two fierce passions: patriotism and education.

Neither of these passions could bring her happiness in Poland. The ideals of democracy affected young Polish people, but the nation had been swallowed by bordering countries: Germany, Austria, and Russia. Warsaw was in the Russian sector. Manya dreaded the inspection days when Russian educators made surprise visits to her school. She was always called on to recite in Russian.

Manya, fascinated by physics apparatus and science experiments, graduated from high school with every possible medal and honor. Now the sixteen-year-old faced a blank wall as far as higher education in Warsaw was concerned. Both Manya and her older sister, Bronya, dreamed of studying medicine in Paris. In the City of Light, Manya might also express some of her political idealism. The sisters began tutoring daughters of wealthy families to earn money to move to Paris.

When she was seventeen, Manya urged Bronya to go Paris and start studying. Manya would continue to work and send her salary to Bronya. "When you are a doctor, you can help me."

"You'd have to wait six years."

Overcoming Bronya's objections, Manya became a governess to a tempestuous ten-year-old. An older sister, Manya's age, became her close friend and made tolerable an unpleasant situation. Soon Manya and the rich young woman were teaching classes together in Polish language and Polish history for peasant children, an activity that was exciting, dangerous, and illegal.

In Paris, Bronya became engaged to a young Polish doctor. They sent for Manya, who arrived in Paris in 1891. For six years she had longed for the hour when she could enroll in the Sorbonne. In the university register, she became for the first time "Marie."

In the community of Polish expatriates, Marie found the home of Bronya and her husband, Dr. Casimir Dluski, joyous and social. At many parties, young Paderewski, a famous composer and president of Poland, played the Dluskis' upright piano. Conversations about medicine, politics, and science kept Marie stimulated and up late. But she needed to study, so she moved to a small attic room and survived on bread, tea, and an occasional egg. In the freezing Parisian winters, she banked the fire to save money and piled all her clothing on her bed.

She passed the master's examination in physics at the head of her class and started to study for a second master's in mathematics. When she told a Polish friend she needed practical laboratory experience, he introduced her to Pierre Curie, a gifted young French scientist.

Pierre, magnetized by the beautiful pale blond Polish woman, who was shy and reserved, was impressed by her brilliance. He tried to talk her out of her revolutionary ideas. "You're knocking your pretty head against a stone wall. Give your energies to science."

Marie responded to his affections and they were married in July 1895. They were poor, and Marie insisted that their wedding be different from other weddings. No white lace gown, no gold ring, no wedding breakfast, no religious ceremony. All they owned in the world were the clothes on their backs and two bicycles, bought the day before the wedding with money sent by a cousin.

Married life was as radiant as the radium they were to discover. She was soon glowingly pregnant. Marie enjoyed keeping house, preparing meals, and studying for her doctorate. She was interested in X rays, which could expose a photographic plate even though the plate was protected by thick, black, lightproof paper.

Thinking only of writing a doctoral dissertation, she worked in a glass-enclosed storeroom full of defunct machinery. She explored the property of radioactivity, not only in uranium but in all known elements. Quickly eliminating seventy-six of the seventy-eight then known, she explored two for radioactivity: uranium and thorium.

Pierre was convinced that her thesis would affect the world of science. But what would be a convenient ore to work with to finish her thesis

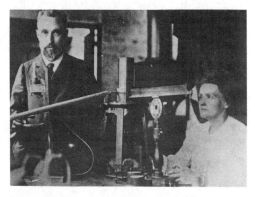

Marie and Pierre recognized that radium could be a weapon in the fight against cancer. *(Photo courtesy of Institute Curie, Paris.)*

project? She decided on Bohemian pitchblende. Where was Marie Curie going to get a ton of pitchblende? An Austrian friend assured her he could have it shipped from Bohemia, and the Curies paid for it from their meager funds.

In the pitchblende she made a discovery that she would not have predicted in her wildest dreams: a new element. Isolating three-tenths of an ounce of pure radium salt from that ton of pitchblende involved hard physical labor, stirring a boiling mass all day long with a heavy iron rod—for forty-eight months. What a thrill for Marie Curie when the substance extracted from pitchblende proved to be a previously unobserved metal.

She called it "polonium"—for the Poland that had aroused such passionate patriotism in her as a young child.

The second unknown element the Curies extracted was the most radioactive substance in the world. Marie called it "radium."

In 1905 Marie completed her dissertation on radioactivity and was granted the degree of doctor of physical science by the University of Paris. As Pierre had predicted, the world of science was affected by her dissertation.

While Marie did not live to see the development of the full resources of atomic energy, the Curies early recognized that radium could be a weapon in the fight against cancer. Had Marie decided to patent the method of extracting radium from uranium ore, she might have become one of the wealthiest women in the world. But she insisted that radium "is for everyone."

In 1903 Pierre and Marie were awarded the Nobel Prize in Physics with Henri Becquerel. Only three years later, the triumph was darkened by tragedy: Pierre Curie was killed by two runaway horses. Marie, now a widow with small children to rear, taught at the University of Paris.

In 1911 Marie was again honored with a Nobel Prize, this time for chemistry.

World War I erupted in 1914, and Marie dedicated herself to French military medical service by equipping an automobile with a portable X-ray machine and a dynamo. At the battlefront, the X rays allowed the doctors to see the exact location of bullets and shell fragments in mutilated and wounded soldiers, averting the need for painful probing.

In 1923 Marie Curie, elected to the French Academy of Medicine, was honored with recognition of the role she took in the discovery of radium and of a new treatment in medicine, "Curietherapy." She died in 1934, a victim of the radioactive substances she had herself discovered.

For most of its editions, the *Encyclopedia Britannica* did not even have a separate entry for Marie Curie, but classified her second to her husband: Curie, Pierre (1869–1906), and Marie (1867–1934), French physicists.

Gerty Radnitz Cori

The first woman to receive a Nobel Prize in Medicine was Dr. Gerty Radnitz Cori. Of Dr. Cori, Rosalyn Yalow wrote: "Consider the history of one woman who had an enormous impact on academic medicine." Gerty Radnitz was born in Prague in 1896, the eldest of three daughters in a Jewish family. Her father, Otto Radnitz, was a chemist and successful owner of several beet-sugar factories.

Graduating at sixteen from a girls' academy with the typical education "appropriate to a woman," she was inspired by an uncle, a professor of pediatrics, to study medicine. To be accepted for medical school, she needed eight years of Latin (she had none), five more years of mathematics, plus physics and chemistry.

Vacationing in the Tyrol the summer after graduation, she met a teacher in the gymnasium in Tetschen who, learning of her plans, began instructing her.

By the end of the summmmer, Gerty Radnitz had mastered three years of Latin. During the next year, she completed all the course work, including math through calculus, passed the examinations, and entered medical school at the University of Prague.

From 1917 to 1919, Gerty was a student assistant in the medical school, fascinated with biochemistry. She began to believe that biochemistry could be the answer to many medical problems.

Gerty Radnitz met Carl F. Cori while they were doing research in immunology. He was tall, fair, good-looking, and shy, but immediately attracted to Gerty, vivacious and brilliant, with red-brown hair and sparkling brown eyes. They shared their vacations mountain climbing and skiing. Shortly after they both received their medical degrees in 1920, they were married.

Gerty became an assistant in the Vienna Children's Hospital until 1922 when the Coris immigrated to the United States. Both Coris worked at the New York State Institute for the Study of Malignant Disease in Buffalo. Carl also taught at the University of Buffalo, and Gerty concentrated on biochemical research.

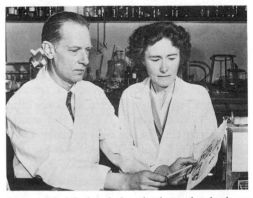

They loved the United States and lost no time in becoming American citizens.

Gerty and Carl Cori worked so closely together that it was difficult to tell where the work of one left off and the other began. They were the third married couple to receive a Nobel Prize in Science. *(Photo courtesy of Washington University, St. Louis, Missouri.)*

In 1931 the two doctors, partners in parenthood and research, were invited to Washington University in St. Louis, Dr. Carl Cori as a professor and Dr. Gerty Cori as a research associate, a lower position. In view of university rules those days, which prohibited hiring both husband and wife in the same department, the university did her a favor. Gerty did not attain full professorship until sixteen years later, after she and her husband jointly received the Nobel Prize in 1947.

They became the third married couple to receive a Nobel Prize in Science. (As we have seen, in 1903 the physics prize went to Pierre and Marie Curie, who shared it with a third French scientist. In 1935 the chemistry prize was awarded to Frederic and Irene Joliot-Curie, daughter of Madame Curie.)

The Coris shared the 1947 Nobel Prize in Physics and Medicine with a third winner, Dr. Bernardo Houssay of Argentina. The Coris made their adopted city of St. Louis proud, and in 1946 they were presented with a gold medallion by the St. Louis Section of the American Chemical Society. Dr. Arthur H. Compton, Nobel Prize winner and chancellor of Washington University, said, "The fame of Carl and Gerty Cori is based upon the reliability of their careful measurements."

In the early years, Carl alone received widespread recognition. Yet they worked so closely together that it was difficult to tell where the work of one left off and the other began. Only after receiving the 1947 Nobel Prize did other honors come Gerty's way: in 1950, the Sugar Research Prize of the National

Academy of Sciences; honorary doctorates from Boston University in 1948, from Smith College in 1949, from Yale in 1951, and from Columbia in 1954.

The work of the Coris in carbohydrate metabolism, especially the discovery of glucose-phosphate, which now bears the name "Corester," was of enormous value in understanding diabetes and brought both Coris many honors.

A fellow scientist at Washington University, Edward A. Doisy, said, "Genius the Coris have. No question about it. But their capacity for hard work has aided that genius to blossom and benefit mankind."

Dorothy Crowfoot Hodgkin

In 1964 Dorothy Hodgkin was the third woman to win the Nobel Prize in Chemistry. Trained as a biochemist, her remarkable discoveries in the X-ray analysis of large molecules led to a knowledge of the penicillin molecule and to the structure of vitamin B12. Dorothy was born in 1910 in Cairo. Her father, John Winter Crowfoot, a classic scholar and archeologist, directed the Egyptian Ministry of Education. Dorothy spent some of her early school vacations on archeological digs in the Near East. Her early dream was to become an archeologist.

Her mother, Grace Mary Crowfoot (called Molly), was the model of a supportive wife, traveling between Africa and England with her husband. She earned an international reputation for her knowledge of Coptic textiles. Educated as a botanist, she drew gorgeous flower illustrations for a book, *Flora,* published in the Sudan.

At the outset of World War I, when Dorothy was four years old, her parents left her and two sisters in England. During the next four years, Dorothy saw her mother only once. An excellent student, she used a chemistry book to do experiments with copper sulfate and alum crystals in school.

When Molly Crowfoot returned to England after the Armistice, she had with her a fourth daughter, Diana. Molly tutored her older daughters, encouraging them to keep notebooks on history, flowers, and birds, and she had them memorize poetry. For the rest of her life, Dorothy recalled and recited with pleasure the poems she learned in those years.

When the family returned to the Sudan, Dorothy learned to prospect for gold. Panning in her backyard, she found a shiny black mineral. Having studied qualitative analysis, she determined it was ilmenite, an iron and titanium mix. With a gift of a surveyors' box of reagents and minerals and a textbook of analytical chemistry, she experimented alone.

Though Dorothy hoped to study at Oxford, she was unqualified to pass entrance exams. Without question, she could do well in chemistry, but she needed a second science. Molly tutored her in botany, and Dorothy passed her entrance exams to Oxford with flying colors.

In 1925 Molly suggested Dorothy study a children's book by W. H. Bragg, *Concerning the Nature of Things*. A line in that book stuck in Dorothy's memory: "Broadly speaking, the discovery of X-rays has increased the keenness of our vision over ten thousand times and we can now 'see' the individual atoms and molecules."

Not only did W. H. Bragg inspire Dorothy, so did his son, who pioneered in studies leading to a famous mathematical formula known as Bragg's law. In 1914 the Braggs, father and son, won the Nobel Prize in Chemistry. Lawrence, only twenty-four, became the youngest Nobel laureate in history.

Though X-ray crystallography was in its infancy, many ladies of leisure in England in the nineteenth century owned chemistry sets. They grew crystals and conducted experiments, an interest regarded as a suitable hobby; however, the pastime led to published research in women's chemistry journals and scientific lectures to feminine crowds. Before going to Oxford, Dorothy spent six months with her father in Jerusalem, where he directed the British School of Archeology. Dorothy, infatuated with archeology, recorded the mosaic floors of Byzantine churches that the Crowfoots helped excavate.

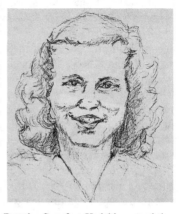

Most of her first year at Oxford, she studied physics. By her second year, Dorothy found crystallography far more challenging than Bragg's little book intimated. Crystallography was like trying to determine the shape of a jungle gym by studying the shadows of its bars; a trial structure had to be determined and later refined.

Dorothy Crowfoot Hodgkin around the time she won the Nobel Prize in Medicine. Later in life, she was badly crippled with arthritis. *(Drawing by Delores Hays Landrum.)*

Dorothy, challenged by the mysteries of chemistry, concentrated on the intricacies of X-ray analysis of large molecules. Archeology would always intrigue her, but chemistry became more than a job: it became a calling.

On a train soon after graduating, she met an old acquaintance, a chemistry professor, A. F. Joseph.

"Why not look up John Desmond Bernal at Cambridge University?" he suggested. "Bernal is studying the use of X-rays to learn about biological crystals, proteins mostly. Isn't that your specialty?"

The encounter proved propitious. Bernal, a visionary scientist strongly in favor of equal opportunities for women scientists, welcomed Dorothy Crowfoot to Cambridge and encouraged her to study for a doctoral degree. She was in seventh heaven, working in Bernal's lab and continuing her research on the earliest X-ray studies of vitamin B1, vitamin D, sex hormones, and protein crystals.

A devoted Aunt Dorothy had subsidized her niece's Oxford education and willingly continued her financial assistance at Cambridge, where Dorothy was being called "the gentle genius."

When Somerville, the women's college at Oxford, offered her a position teaching chemistry, she refused at first, reluctant to leave Bernal's lab. She concentrated on solid cyclic alcohols found in plant and animal tissues and studied interesting crystals that had been sent to Bernal from around the world. She credited all her subsequent work to "looking at crystals with Bernal."

When Somerville made a second offer allowing her to stay on at Cambridge for another year and then move to Somerville, she could complete her doctoral research for a Ph.D. before assuming teaching responsibilities.

She achieved miracles in two years at Cambridge, earning her doctorate, then studying the X-ray diffraction of crystals of the digestive enzyme peptide, the work that won her the Nobel Prize.

Arriving at Oxford, she found she was the only woman on the faculty. She felt lonely in the early years. Women were excluded from membership or attendance at the weekly symposium about current research in chemistry, but she could attend general sessions and never missed any. Studying the men's work on sterols, especially cholesterol, she found much of the previously accepted formulas incorrect. Such a finding did not make her popular.

On a bitter winter day in 1934, the joints of her hands hurt and were so inflamed and tender that Dorothy had difficulties with her experiments. Her parents insisted on taking her to a London specialist, who diagnosed rheumatoid arthritis, "a severe case." There was little to do for this disease before cortisone became available. Years later, in 1978, the famed English artist Henry Moore made a drawing of her crippled hands.

Dorothy never complained of pain. Astonishingly her handwriting remained legible and lovely for the rest of her life.

For Dorothy, at twenty-seven, 1937 was a stellar year. She was awarded her doctorate and met Thomas L. Hodgkin, a Quaker who shared Dorothy's liberal sympathies. Instant fireworks.

Thomas came from a family as extraordinary as the Crowfoots, sharing their sense of social responsibility and intellectual curiosity. One of Thomas's ancestors, Luke Howard, is considered the father of meteorology. Thomas's cousin, Alan Hodgkin, received the Nobel Award in Physiology and Medicine only a year before Dorothy won that honor.

Dorothy and Thomas were married in 1937 and honeymooned for two months in the south of France. Theirs was a true love match, but they had to be content with togetherness only on alternate weekends, since Dorothy continued teaching at Oxford and Thomas worked for the Friends Service Council in Stoke-on-Trent.

Dorothy and Thomas's three children had careers of their own: Luke taught mathematics at the University of Algiers, Elizabeth taught in a Zambian girls school, and Toby volunteered as a social worker in India. They could boast that they had Nobel Prize winners on both sides of the family.

Much of the success of this two-career family belonged to Thomas, who had enormous respect for his wife's career. He took charge of the children's evenings when Dorothy returned to her lab. However, Dorothy remembered a time when her son wanted her to hear his first violin lesson at the time she was to be interviewed for a grant from the Rockefeller Foundation. During the questioning, she glanced at her watch, explained the situation, and asked to be excused. The interviewer was charmed.

Did Dorothy ever feel guilty about her role as mother? She saw her children develop independence and self-esteem. Moreover, she was grateful that during her three pregnancies she had surprising relief from the pain of her rheumatoid arthritis and easier use of her hands. Eventually, she found some improvement when the discovery of the hormone cortisone reduced the inflammation of arthritis. In her lab, she zipped her crippled feet into ankle-high slippers.

By 1940 Britain was at war, and Dorothy was finishing her research on cholesterol. After penicillin was discovered by Alexander Flemming, Ernst Cain, and Howard Florey, Dorothy requisitioned crystalline specimens of salts as soon as they became available. She began experiments with a research team to determine the position of the sulfur atoms in the crystal lattice.

In 1942 information on the structure of penicillin was vital because large quantities of the antibiotic were needed for the war wounded. Dorothy conducted research on the recalcitrant molecule with cobalt atom heart, essential to human life. Working in a cluttered, dingy basement, with no heat, beneath the university museum, she had to climb a precarious ladder to a gallery, carrying delicate crystals in her arthritic hands.

Her Oxford lab, as crowded and cluttered as her large rented house, was informal and often considered "bizarre." Everyone called her "Dorothy," something rare for a European professor. She encouraged women scientists, who considered her the cleverest woman in Europe. Some of the researchers' calculations for electron density maps were being done on electrical punched-card machines. The magnitude of the data seemed endless.

The Hodgkins were world travelers; Dorothy had been to China, the Soviet Union, and the United States. She had been elected a fellow of the Royal Society and received their Royal and Copley Medals. Awarded the Order of Merit in 1965, she was the only woman so honored since Florence Nightingale. She was the first Wolfson Research Professor of the Royal Society and was invited to be a member of the prestigious American Academy of Arts and Sciences.

Thomas lectured at Northwestern University in Illinois in 1957 and at the Institute of Islamic Studies at McGill University in Montreal, Quebec, in 1958.

Dr. Hodgkin, on her last night in London before flying to Sweden for the Nobel ceremonies, addressed the Swedish Academy of Science. She spoke of an Arabian party in Ghana, where her hosts had advised her that when you reply in Arabic to congratulations on a happy event, such as the birth of a son or the marriage of a daughter, you say, "May this happen also to you." And then, this modest, beautiful woman beamed. "May this happen also to you."

In Stockholm, Dorothy Hodgkin spoke on behalf of the 1964 Nobel Prize winners to an assembly of Swedish students. She said she was chosen to address them "as one woman of our group, a position which I hope very much will not be so very uncommon in the future that it will call for any comment or distinctions of this kind, as more and more women carry out research in the same way as men." Eager to stand up for the poor, the oppressed, and the cause of peace, she said she spoke "as a countrywoman of Tom Paine who wrote an early book on the rights of man, from whom the declaration of human rights derived."

Dorothy created two glowing reputations: one under her maiden name, Crowfoot, and one under her married name, Hodgkin. Around the world, scientists were amazed that the Crowfoot of penicillin fame and the Hodgkin of B12 fame were one and the same person. She carried on with a wizardry of intellectual unraveling, quiet enthusiasm, and an elegance of achievement until her death in 1994.

Barbara McClintock

Barbara McClintock, a botanist who shied from publicity, won the 1983 Nobel Prize for her discovery that genes could move around on plant chromosomes, causing changes in heredity. Hers was the first Nobel Prize in Medicine given for work originally done in higher plants.

Ordinarily, this prize, worth about $190,000 in 1983, recognizes work in medicine, animal biology, or microbiology. McClintock was the first woman ever to win an unshared Nobel Prize in medicine or physiology. She was the third woman to win an unshared Nobel Prize in Science.

After learning of her award, Dr. McClintock, eighty-one, went out to pick walnuts along a wooded path near her home at Cold Spring Harbor Laboratory, Long Island, New York. Later, she observed, "The prize is such an extraordinary honor. It might seem unfair, however, to reward a person for having so much pleasure, over the years, asking the maize plant to solve specific problems and then watching its responses."

Dr. McClintock, a lifelong breaker of rules, enrolled in Cornell at seventeen over her mother's objections. Barbara did not remember where she learned about college or even how she determined to go to college. Her father was overseas in the army and the family had little money.

In autumn, her father returned from Europe and convinced Barbara's mother that their daughter deserved to go on for higher education. Agreeably, her mother called a friend whose daughter went to Cornell and asked when the semester began.

She learned that students whose name began with M were registering the following Tuesday. Because Barbara had a job, her mother took over the task of trying to get her daughter's high school records. She got nothing.

Barbara, undaunted, caught a train to Ithaca. First off, she confidently rented a room. Everyone else registering had school records. The registrar asked Barbara, "How do you expect to get in?"

Through a stroke of inexplicable luck, she managed to get her class assignments. "I went to zoology and was entranced at the very first lecture." That enthusiasm stayed with her all through college.

Barbara attended Cornell University College of Agriculture because tuition was free. Knowing that family finances were critical, she hoped to finish college as quickly as possible. She signed up for an incredible number of courses. If she dropped out because she didn't like the course, she got a Z. By the time she was a junior, her records were covered with Zs.

In contrast to her solitary childhood, she had an active social life. The women's freshman class elected her president. She made friends with an intellectual group of women. She found her Jewish friends particularly stimulating. Drawn to these women, she enjoyed their differences and even spent time learning to read Yiddish. Shocked that they were discriminated against and refused membership in sororities, she developed a distinct distaste for honorary societies. In later life, she only joined scientific organizations because she felt obligated.

Long before the style became fashionable, she had her hair cut short. Earning money by working in the cornfields, she decided she wanted knickers and had a tailor make up "plus fours" for her. Although she dated several men and had an emotional attachment to some, none of them were scientists.

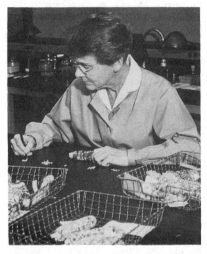

Barbara McClintock in 1944 at her workbench. *(Photo courtesy of Carnegie Institution, Washington, D.C.)*

She told her biographer, Evelyn Fox Keller, "I never could understand marriage; I never went through the experience of requiring it."

She was barred from majoring in plant breeding, on the ground of "feminine sensibilities." Not daunted, she wormed her way into genetics through the ladylike auspices of botany.

In her junior year at Cornell, she did so well in genetics, the professor urged her to take a graduate course in the subject. Accepted in graduate school, she won fellowships to study genetics of corn. In 1927 she became Barbara McClintock, Ph.D., with an assistant professorship.

Her fellow scientists considered her research a little crazy. Fortunately, Marcus Rhoades, a young graduate student who was to become a leading geneticist, arrived at Cornell to study for his Ph.D. Determined to study maize, he was excited by Dr. McClintock's research. He immediately understood what others regarded as controversial. Rhoades provided Barbara with much-needed intellectual companionship.

From 1929 to 1931, McClintock published nine papers detailing her research in maize chromosomes. This was a time that her biographer called "the Golden Age of maize cyto-genetics." McClintock inspired Rhoades and other geneticists. Dr. Rhoades later observed, "I used her papers as teaching models of scientific clarity and rigor. I've known a lot of famous scientists, but the only one I thought really was a genius was McClintock."

Marcus Rhoades marveled that Barbara could look at a cell under the microscope and see so much. She responded, "Well, you know, when I look at a cell, I get down in that cell and look around!"

In 1933 Dr. McClintock received a Guggenheim Fellowship to go to Germany. Many of her closest friends were Jewish. In Germany she was horrified at the political climate and hastened to return to Cornell. Now a slim boyish figure with a boy's haircut, she was unemployed and depressed about the world situation.

Over the years at Cornell, Barbara McClintock was kept from tenure because she was a woman. From 1931 to 1933, she divided her time between the University of Missouri, California Institute of Technology, and Cornell. Her first offer of a faculty position came from Lewis Stadler at the University of Missouri in Columbia. She completed her work on ring chromosomes and investigated the way that broken chromosomes tend to reanneal. Even the successful research at Missouri did not ensure promotions.

Having stifled her dislike for organizations, she joined the Genetics Society of America and in 1939 was elected vice president. At the outbreak of World War II, Barbara left Missouri and was at loose ends. She was invited to Cold Spring Harbor for the summer and then offered a one-year appointment.

For the next forty years, McClintock lived and worked alone at the Cold Spring Harbor Laboratory as a scientist of the Carnegie Institute of Washington. Biographer Evelyn Fox Keller describes McClintock's solitary work at Cold Spring Harbor. "Each spring she plants her corn, judiciously fertilizing the budding kernels according to a carefully worked out plan of genetic courses, watches the plants grow over the summer, and spends the long quiet winters analyzing the results." Her career may paraphrase the little red hen that asked in vain, "Who will help me plant my corn?"

In 1970 McClintock became an independent Distinguished Service Member of the Carnegie Institute. Her studies of color changes in maize led to her findings of mobile genetic elements, also known as "jumping genes," on chromosomes. For years, her experiments were belittled. Finally they were accepted as helpful to understanding human diseases (such as cancer) and how bacteria can become resistant to drugs.

In awarding Dr. McClintock the Nobel Prize, the committee said she had been "far ahead of the enormous genetic discoveries of recent decades, including that of the structure of DNA."

The committee pointed to the historical similarity between McClintock's lone situation and that of Gregor Mendel who, studying the garden pea a century earlier, discovered basic principles of genetics. Both scientists were so far ahead of their time that their discoveries were neither appreciated nor recognized until the principles were rediscovered by other geneticists decades later.

The Nobel Prize capped a long list of honors and awards for McClintock. In 1984 she was still working on maize genetics with what her longtime friend Marcus Rhoades described as "her boundless energy; her complete devotion to science; her originality and ingenuity; her quick wit and high intelligence." McClintock died in 1992.

Rita Levi-Montalcini

Rita Levi-Montalcini, born in Turin, Italy, in 1909, came from an upper-middle-class, educated Jewish family. With her twin sister and the rest of her family, Rita went into hiding in Italy during the Second World War. Their lives were constantly in danger, and they experienced the heavy hand of fascism.

Levi-Montalcini became the fourth woman to win a Nobel Prize in Medicine, sharing the honor in 1986 with her American colleague, Dr. Stanley Cohen, an American biochemist and researcher. Levi-Montalcini and Cohen received the award for contributing to the understanding and potential treatment of cancerous tumors, senility, and other diseases.

In her biography, Dr. Levi-Montalcini recounts how Dr. Cohen (she called him "Stan") limped into the lab at Washington University in St. Louis on a winter day in 1953. (He had been a polio victim as a child.) At once, he impressed her with his courage and modesty. They worked harmoniously together.

"Rita," Stan said, "you and I are good, but together we are wonderful."

And so it proved to be. In a laboratory charged with enthusiasm and anxious expectations, she "lived the six most intense, productive years of my life."

As a feisty young woman, Rita was unqualified for college because of a typical Italian girlhood education. Observing that women always played a subordinate role, she made up her mind she would not be a wife and mother.

Twenty years old when she applied for admission to medical school, she was required to study Greek, Latin, and advanced mathematics with tutors. A younger cousin, Eugenia, enthusiastically joined Rita's project, and both women passed exams to be accepted to the University of Turin. Eventually, Rita earned her M.D. in neurology.

Unlike Eugenia, Rita made few friends. Years later, one of her fellow students remarked that when Rita was young, she was "just impossible, a kind of squid ready to squirt ink at anybody."

When Rita was forced to resign from her university position because she was Jewish, she promptly set up a small laboratory in her bedroom and resumed research into how periphery affected the development of the nervous system in its nascent stages. Six months later, when Mussolini declared war on England and France, Allied planes bombed Turin. The family fled to a small house near Asti.

Her instruments, glassware, and chemical reagents necessary for her project were similar to the ones that her nineteenth-century predecessors had used. She continued experiments on eggs with chick embryos, begging farmers for such eggs "for her babies." She explained to the farmers they were "more nutritious."

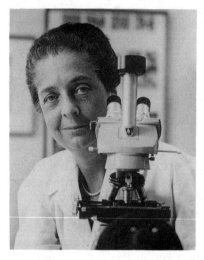

On July 25, 1943, Mussolini fled with the royal family and fascist generals from Italy. German tanks were parked outside the Turin railway station. For non-Aryans, there was no choice but to go into hiding to save their lives from barbarian hordes invading the country. Rita's family fled to Florence and remained in hiding until the Allies arrived in 1944.

From September 1944 to May 1945, she served as a doctor for the allies in a refugee camp. Night and day, trucks brought dying old people, women, and children who had abdominal typhus and cholera.

The war ended in northern Italy in April 1945, and the family could return to Turin. Rita went back to working as an assistant to her lifetime teacher, Professor Giuseppe Levi, at the university. He warned her that her research could ruin her reputation and his, but she persisted and turned established theory on its head.

Rita Levi-Montalcini, Nobel Prize winner and author of *In Praise of Imperfection: My Life and Work.* (Photo courtesy of Washington University, St. Louis, Missouri.)

In 1946 she was invited to come to Washington University in St. Louis, Missouri, by Viktor Hamburger to spend a semester in the department of zoology. He had read one of her papers on the mechanisms governing the effects of peripheral tissues and the nerve fibers that innervate them. He wanted to collaborate with her to investigate the problem.

At Washington University, she admired the relaxed attitudes between professors and students. She enjoyed seeing students relishing their classes and research. After years of observing the strict rules in Italian university libraries, she liked seeing American students studying in the library with their feet on the desk.

Levi-Montalcini had expected to be in the United States a few months but remained for twenty years. She was proud to become a naturalized U.S. citizen, holding dual Italian and American citizenship.

In 1952 she arrived in Rio de Janeiro where an old friend, Hertha Meyer, had established a tissue culture laboratory at the Institute of Biophysics. Levi-Montalcini, eager to join her research, had brought with her two white mice spying through the holes of a tiny cardboard box.

In 1986, with the king and queen present at a ceremony in Sweden, Rita Levi-Montalcini received the Noble Prize for her work in nerve growth factor (NGF), the first of a family of endogenous specific growth factors. Thanks to the simplicity and clarity of the bioassay, experiments proved that the tumors released a growth factor in the culture medium.

In 1988 Basic Books published her autobiography, *In Praise of Imperfection* (translated by Luigi Attardi, Sloan Foundation Science Series), a personal account of the gifted daughter of a "free thinking" family. The autobiography reveals a capacity for genius to blossom and to benefit humankind.

A woman of unyielding determination, she surmounted all obstacles to become a doctor and a successful medical researcher. Critical of the conventional attitudes of male superiority, she was an Italian woman with a dazzling, indomitable spirit. In 2000, she still pursued research at the Institute of Neurobiology's National Council of Research in Rome, Italy.

Gertrude Elion

Among the uneasy careers of female physicians and scientists, Gertrude B. Elion's life enfolds a pattern of great pleasure in creativity and success in research.

The woman who helped develop some of the most renowned drugs of the twentieth century was turned down repeatedly for research positions because the organizations had never had a woman in the lab.

"They thought I would be a distraction," Gertrude Elion recalled at the Nobel Prize ceremonies in Stockholm in 1988. Elion, the only woman on the stage, wore a royal blue chiffon gown, striking a note of brilliance among the starched white shirts and formal black suits of the other recipients. Her colleague in the honors, George Herbert Hitchings, eighty-three, also stood out as the oldest Nobel recipient.

With Britain's Sir James Black, Drs. Elion and Hitchings were receiving the 1988 Nobel Prize in Physiology or Medicine for pioneering research in medications to treat some of humankind's most threatening diseases. Her award was especially noteworthy since Nobel Prizes usually honored academic scientists. Such recognition to someone working in the pharmaceutical industry was rare. So reluctant is the Nobel Committee to reward commercial research that the prize did not come until thirty years after most of the discoveries.

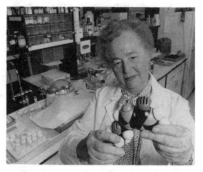

Gertrude Elion: "Research [is] an unraveling of mysteries." (*Photo courtesy of Burroughs Wellcome.*)

Hitchings and Elion collaborated for forty years, demonstrating differences in nucleic acid metabolism between normal human cells, cancer cells, protozoa, bacteria, and viruses. They developed a series of drugs to combat leukemia and tissue rejection in kidney transplant patients. They studied drugs that would block the processes of growth and reproduction of cancer cells and noxious organisms without damaging normal human cells, work that had enormous significance in cancer and antiviral research.

Elion, born in 1918, was fifteen when her grandfather died of cancer. Despairing, Elion felt a "need to do something," and she decided on a career in an age when women rarely set their prime sights on a profession. An excellent student in high school, she was interested in all her subjects, especially biology and chemistry. "I was very good at dissection."

Appointed to her high school honor society, she was asked by career guidance interviewers about her goals. She replied she did not want to teach because she didn't have the patience; she wanted to be a scientist. "It took me years to understand why they laughed at that answer. I came to realize how ironic it was. You can't do research if you are not patient."

In 1937 Elion graduated summa cum laude from Hunter College in New York and began working in a laboratory of the New York Hospital School of Nursing. She later accepted an unpaid position with an organic chemist, who eventually paid her $20 a month. From this meager sum she saved enough to study at New York University. The job market was bleak when she earned a master's degree in 1941. A two-hour interview concluded with rejection; they would not hire a woman.

For a year and a half, Elion worked as a food analyst for Quaker Maid Company, testing the acidity of pickles and checking berries slated for jam to make sure they weren't moldy.

With the outbreak of the Second World War, a labor shortage presented Elion with an opportunity at Johnson & Johnson, a company embarking on pharmaceutical research. When the vice president who had hired her was fired, she was again out of a job.

Fate intervened when Elion's father, a dentist, brought home a free sample of Empirin, an aspirin produced by Burroughs Wellcome, then in Tuckahoe, New York. Perhaps Burroughs Wellcome would have an opening.

On a Saturday morning in June 1944, the twenty-six-year-old Elion, wearing her best suit, took a train from the Bronx where she lived with her parents. At Tuckahoe, a woman working for Dr. Hitchings urged him not to hire Elion because she was "too well dressed." ("Why wouldn't you wear your best suit for an interview?" Elion was still asking more than four decades later.)

In an interview years later, Dr. Hitchings remembered that Elion hoped to receive a salary of $50 a week. Impressed by Elion's intelligence and enthusiasm, he thought she was worth at least that.

The Tuckahoe lab had two floors. Hitchings worked on one and Elion on the other. Scientists ran up and down the stairs to exchange ideas. Elion was happy; the work was always collaborative and uncompetitive. Her immersion in her research became her lifestyle.

When Elion began working with Hitchings, he was doing most of the cancer research at Burroughs Wellcome. With the very first cancer drug on which Elion collaborated, they "struck gold." Hitchings's lab, when Elion joined the company, was studying nucleic acids, the basic chemical structures for animals.

One of the nucleic acids, purine, became Elion's specialty. "My whole life has been involved in purines, the parent substance of the uric-acid group of compounds," she later told her university students.

Her first discovery was a purine compound called 6-mercaptopurine, an antileukemia drug. She synthesized the drug in the late 1950s. Animal tests showed that the compound inhibited the growth of tumors.

Sent to Sloan-Kettering Institute, the compound proved effective in clinical trials on children with acute leukemia. The director of Sloan-Kettering gave the history of the effective drug to Walter Winchell, a radio journalist. His bombastic announcement resulted in hundreds of letters pouring into the lab, begging for the drug that continues to be a prime treatment for leukemia.

"I can't think of anything more exciting than seeing a drug you worked on being used," Elion said in an interview. She experienced this satisfaction repeatedly. In the early 1960s, she synthesized Immuran (azathioprine), an immunosuppressant making kidney transplants possible. She tested Zyloprim, discovered in 1966, as a possible cure for the age-old scourge of gout. Her experiments with a drug for Leishmaniasis, a tropical disease, led to World Health Organization testing.

For a decade, Elion's laboratory studies focused on Zovirax, an antiherpes agent. She found that a substance released by the herpes virus actually activates the drug used to treat the disease. The next logical research project for Burroughs Wellcome was to join the challenge of finding a cure for AIDS.

When Elion found love, the man she expected to marry died of subacute bacterial endocarditis. For a long time she had to fight her grief. Her discoveries became the offspring she had hoped to have. She would not say which was her favorite. "Each discovery at the time is a highlight. I feel like a mother to some of the compounds."

In fact, when someone said something derogatory about one of her projects, she came to its defense "like a lioness."

Though she channeled her passions into research, she admitted she would have liked to have had a family. Greatly loved and admired by her many nieces and nephews, she treated eleven members of her family to a trip to Stockholm for the Nobel ceremonies!

In her retirement, Elion enthusiastically became adjunct professor at Duke University and University of North Carolina–Chapel Hill. From 1983 until her death in 1999, she was a mentor for medical and graduate students in the neuro-oncology and pediatric bone marrow transplant programs. Her students called her "Trudy" and remembered her as a born teacher. She delighted in the achievements of her younger associates. During her years at Duke, she published more than twenty-five papers with her students and modestly refused to put her name on published papers simply because the work had been done in her lab. This attitude was not a common approach in science. *

According to Michael Colvin of the Duke Comprehensive Cancer Center, Durham, North Carolina, "Faculty and staff remembered her as a brilliant, determined scientist." Though she could never get away from her lab long enough to earn a Ph.D., she was awarded honorary doctorates by twenty-five universities.

She translated German patents and held forty-five patents of her own. In 1985 she received the North Carolina Distinguished Chemist Award. One of her most cherished honors was serving on the National Cancer Advisory Board.

In 1991 Gertrude Elion became the first woman to be voted into the Inventors Hall of Fame, a nonprofit organization in Akron, Ohio. Cited for pioneering research at the Burrough Wellcome Company, at seventy-three Elion was delighted to be enshrined among the Bells and Edisons. "I'm happy to be the first woman," she said, "but I doubt I'll be the last."

Science, Vol. 284, May 28, 1999, p. 1480.

Note: Today women scientists are finding rewarding research positions in the pharmaceutical industry. Determined women have overcome prejudice in the fields that traditionally belonged to men—science, mathematics, and medicine. Whether women can make great contributions is no longer in doubt now that they are offered the resources to achieve their goals thanks to new attitudes in society.

Christiane Nusslein-Volhard

In 1995 Tubingen, a beautiful German village, celebrated the award of the Nobel Prize in Medicine to Christiane Nusslein-Volhard (age fifty-two). Sharing the award were Eric Wieschaus (age forty-eight) of Princeton and Edward B. Lewis (age seventy-seven) of the California Institute of Technology, Pasadena.

Other biologists in the 1990s were working at reducing the problem of how a simple one-celled egg gives rise to the complexity of a complete animal.

Taking an opposite approach, Nusslein-Volhard, director of research at the Max Planck Institute for Development Biology, was studying fruit flies. She wanted to understand the intricate unfurling of an egg into an organism. Working with her colleagues, she hoped to discover the genetic script that causes the orderly, reliable, marvelous miracle of creating a new living thing.

The work that won the Nobel Prize may reveal not only answers to the basic riddles of human development, but may also shed light on problems of well-being and life-threatening diseases such as cancer.

Why are so many babies—as many as one in twenty-eight—born with a birth defect? Why do half of all pregnancies end in miscarriages? Do miscarriages result from flaws in the genes that orchestrate development? Do these bad genes cause cancers?

Nusslein-Volhard and Wieschaus first published results in 1980, identifying key genes for making a fertilized fruit fly egg develop into a segmented embryo. The two scientists found that the genes create the first broad strokes of what the embryo is going to look like.

In California, working independently, Dr. Lewis published a paper in 1978 explaining how master switch genes control development of organs in specific body segments and how a flaw in the "master control genes" can produce extra wings or legs in fruit flies.

The Nobel Prize winners discovered that such principles apply as well to humans, and counterparts of the fruit fly genes have been found in people. Nusslein-Volhard's determination to learn how a pregnancy goes swimmingly and results in a normal full-term baby led to a Nobel Prize.

Christiane Nusslein-Volhard, one of very few women directors of German laboratories, with her "fly group" propelled the mysteries of the fruit fly, *Drosophila melanogaster*, down to the molecular level.

Mothering and encouraging her gifted staff, she drew the attention of scientists throughout the world who had pinned their experiments and hopes on zebra fish, a small aquarium species that breeds quickly and produces large, transparent embryos. For five years the group worked in Tubingen to learn to run a fish colony. The aquarium required absolutely clean water, and the fish had to have a diet of fruit fly larvae. Night and day, the "fly group" worried about the care of flies; some carried a jar of flies in a pocket or purse everywhere. Nusslein-Volhard's work yielded some 1,300 mutants from 1.2 million embryos, producing a dazzling number of defects.

"Public fear about gene research on embryos is erroneous," she said. "No one yet fully understands the genes that make humans wiser, more beautiful, or even what makes blue eyes. My discoveries help mankind become wiser, understand biology better, and comprehend how life functions."

When Nusslein-Volhard shifted her focus from the time-honored fruit fly to the common zebra fish, Eric Wieschaus said, "It was a difficult and challenging thing to do."

The zebra fish, an oddly aberrant tiny striped animal, breeds rapidly and produces a large brood. Its embryos develop outside the mother. It is transparent, so scientists watch the heart, brain, and other organs develop. These fish may inform scientists about the shaping of structures and mechanisms specific to vertebrates—a complex nervous system, blood vessels, or kidneys.

In the 1980s, the elite Max Planck Society, an independent but largely government-funded agency operating more than fifty research institutes throughout Germany, presented a bleak picture for women's participation in scientific research.

Among more than 200 research directors, only two were women. The concept that a woman has no business outside of home and family died hard in Germany. *Kinder, küche, kirche* (children, kitchen, church) seemed written in stone.

Janni, as Nusslein-Volhard is known by friends and family, admitted to Jennifer Ackerman, an author writing a book on biological kinships between humans and other species, that she experienced "loneliness, doing things in a solitary way."

Janni was the second of five children, growing up in Frankfurt. In high school, she was fascinated by biology. No one noticed. Everyone in her family painted, and they were passionate about artistic achievements. Science was regarded as insignificant. Her grandmother was an artist; her father and two of her siblings were architects. At the University of Tubingen, surrounded by the Hohentubingen castle, the Neckar River, and medieval half-timbered houses, Janni studied gene transcription in bacteria. With a postdoctoral at the University of Basel in 1975 studying the development of the fruit fly, she found it exquisitely exciting to observe the flies grow and change. Men in the department expected little of a woman, but she soon became obsessed and, indeed, an expert in fruit fly genetics and inventing new systems for research.

German students tend to complete their education at a more leisurely pace

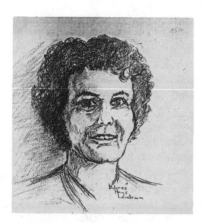

than students elsewhere. Many complete a Ph.D. after the age of thirty. Women, who at that time of life might want to start and raise a family, find it almost impossible to do scientific research requiring twelve-hour days, including weekends. Many of Germany's most prominent women scientists, including Nusslein-Volhard, decided not to have children. About day care in Germany, Dr. Nusslein-Volhard observed in 1990, "You can't get it even if you pay."

In Tubingen in 1991, geneticist Maria Leptin had her first child. She carried the baby to the lab and he slept in her office. At the end of the year, Leptin hired a nanny who, at the last moment, reneged. Leptin teamed up with a neurobiologist who needed child care. While the Max Planck Society refused to use government funds to pay for a facility, Nusslein-

Dr. Christiane Nusslein-Volhard provided knowledge on principles of master switch and master control genes and human development. In 1995 she shared the Nobel Prize in Medicine with two American scientists. *(Drawing by Delores Hays Landrum.)*

Volhard volunteered to pay with one of her scientific prizes. The Tubingen city council supplemented contributions.

The daycare center opened in spring 1992 with twelve children. Because Leptin's husband's work required commuting between Tubingen and Cambridge, England, he was unable to give his wife any help. But the daycare center was so successful it led to the Max Planck Society subsidizing lab-based Tubingen child care and later some nurseries elsewhere.

Dominique Ferrandon, who did his fly research for a doctorate under the tutelage of Dr. Nusslein-Volhard, said she is unstinting in supporting her staff and students.

"Janni is strong and determined," according to Nancy Hopkins, a biologist at Massachusetts Institute of Technology. Biologists claim Nusslein-Volhard is "the most important developmental biologist of the second half of the twentieth century . . . Perhaps, of all time." Other scientists who know the Nobel Prize winner said her work with Wieschaus "is an absolute triumph of pure genetics and pure visual examination. By studying the whole embryo from the outside, they deduced what the genes were doing on the inside.

"We owe Nusslein-Volhard a huge debt. Her zebra fish mutants provide a fantastic system for studying the process of blood formation and critical insights into human disease. The medical applications of her work please Nusslein-Volhard, but it is the very effort of what mutants reveal about development as a whole that excites her most."

Rosalyn Yalow

Among women who have had the greatest impact on career attitudes of the younger generation is Dr. Rosalyn Yalow, who shared the Nobel Prize in Medicine in 1977 with Dr. Roger C. Guillemin of the Salk Institute and Dr. Andrew V. Schally of the Veterans Administration Hospital in New Orleans. The Nobel Prize in Medicine honored these Americans for opening new vistas within biological and medical research in radioimmunossay (RIA), an extremely sensitive analytical technique. Their discoveries revealed that the elevated blood sugar in adult diabetes is due to some unknown factor interfering with the action of insulin and not to insulin deficiency.

The RIA studies also helped determine if the lack of growth in children is due to an inadequate amount of growth hormone or if excessive steroid production by the adrenal gland is due to a tumor of the gland or a message from an overactive pituitary. RIA has also been used to detect drug abuse of heroin, methadone, and LSD. In addition RIA may determine if blood used for transfusion is contaminated with a virus that causes a liver infection. Dr. Yalow believes the technique will find increasing applications in diagnosing infectious diseases.

Born in 1921 in New York City, Yalow always lived and worked there, except for three and a half years when she was a graduate student at the University of Illinois. Her earliest memories were of being a "stubborn, determined child." Her mother rejoiced that Rosalyn was bent on socially acceptable choices.

Her parents were first-generation immigrants whose formal education had ended in elementary school. Even as a youngster, Rosalyn had her mind set on a career in science. An early and avid reader, she was encouraged by a high school teacher of chemistry. Other fine teachers at New York City's Hunter College, an all-women's school, helped her realize that physics was an exciting subject.

"It seemed," observed Dr. Yalow in retrospect, "that every major physics experiment brought a Nobel Prize." She felt inspired by Eve Curie's biography of her mother, Madame Marie Curie.

The only job Yalow could find in her senior year at Hunter College was as a secretary, sharpening pencils and taking dictation at Columbia University's College of Physicians and Surgeons. She had been told she could forget graduate school; she'd never be accepted in physics. But she received a teaching fellowship in physics at the University of Illinois. She wasted no time tearing up her steno books.

Yalow had been the first physics major ever to graduate from Hunter College. In 1941, she was the only woman among 400 faculty members of the College of Engineering. On the first day of graduate school at the University of Illinois, she met her future husband, Aaron Yalow, later professor of physics at Cooper Union in New York City.

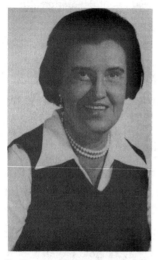

Dr. Rosalyn Yalow was inspired to greatness by Marie Curie. *(Photo courtesy of Rosalyn Yalow.)*

At the University of Illinois, she audited two undergraduate courses to compensate for any possible neglected areas of physics. For credit, she took three graduate courses while teaching freshman physics. Like most teaching assistants, she had no teaching experience. She took time to observe in the classroom of an instructor who had a reputation as an excellent teacher.

When war broke out in 1941, Yalow taught army and navy students pouring into college, while continuing her graduate courses and experiments. She was encouraged by her thesis director, Dr. Maurice Goldhaber, and his wife, Dr. Gertrude Goldhaber, a distinguished physicist in her own right. Gertrude Goldhaber could hold no university position because of nepotism rules, Yalow remembered.

A leading medical physicist, Dr. Edith Quimby, later allowed Dr. Yalow to work in the laboratory of the College of Physicians and Surgeons as a volunteer, studying the medical application of radioisotopes. This led to a part-time position as a consultant at the Bronx Veterans Administration Hospital in 1947, while she continued teaching full-time at Hunter College (1946–1950). In spring 1950, a twenty-two-year partnership with Dr. Solomon A. Berson began that lasted until he died in 1972. Dr. Yalow grieved that he did not survive to share the Nobel Prize with her, as he surely would have had he lived.

Dr. Berson had left the laboratory in 1968 to be chair of the Department of Medicine at the Mount Sinai School of Medicine. After Dr. Berson's untimely death, Rosalyn Yalow asked that their laboratory be designated the Solomon A. Berson Research Laboratory "so that his name will continue to be on my papers as long as I publish."

Aaron and Rosalyn Yalow had a two-career marriage and two children, Benjamin and Elanna. Even after the children were born, Rosalyn Yalow never felt any guilt about her career. She was an involved mother and often chaperoned her children's school activities.

In 1977 when Yalow won the Nobel Prize in Medicine, her mother was in her nineties. "I wish my father could have lived to see this," Dr. Yalow mused. "He died in 1959, just when I started to win awards. He would have been so proud of me."

Dr. Rosalyn Yalow observed, "We like to believe that a young woman starting her professional career would find it easier today. . . . The view of women's roles in society which was prevalent in my generation is gradually changing."

A Future Nobel Prize Winner?

Who will be the future Nobel Prize winner to deal with the tremendous potential of stem cell research? By 2001, this research had begun to reveal that stem cell research shows the possibility of improving and lengthening human life, and dealing with such debilitating problems as Alzheimer's and Parkinson's, cancer and diabetes. And particularly the anguish of infertility.

Most thoughtful citizens recognize the pain of childless couples who want a family. Support is widespread for the use of frozen embryos that would otherwise be discarded by fertility clinics. While doctors continue to pursue every research alternative to the use of embryonic stem cells, viable frozen embryos should be more readily available to help infertile couples realize their hopes.

The federal government would be expected to ensure that no one would receive payment for such embryos.

The annals of medicine are replete with stories of opposition to birth control, heart transplants, blood transfusions, and in vitro fertilization. The opposition to abortion has turned violent, though we read daily about mothers who beat or mistreat, drown, or abandon their children in the most dire situations.

Thousands of mothers owe their sanity to having aborted an unwanted child. Thousands of patients owe their lives to medical research and millions more could benefit from life saving stem cell research.

9

Women's Proper Place:
Our Biological Selves

Author Maria Manes observed, "The beautiful difference of our biological selves will not diminish this mutual fusion. It should indeed flower, expand; blow the mind as well as the flesh, so that men and women can both breathe free."

Among the many women doctors who wrote autobiographies were Rosalie Slaughter Morton and Beatrice Bishop Berle. Both women gloried in their lives as physicians. The lives of such emancipated women offer insights into the extraordinary courage they needed to be a doctor in the nineteenth century.

Rosalie Slaughter Morton

At the turn of the nineteenth century, Dr. Rosalie Slaughter Morton predicted the struggle for equality would be won, that men and women released from guilt or blame or hate could use the best of each other's qualities to cherish life and love.

In 1937 when Rosalie Slaughter Morton published *A Woman Surgeon*, she wrote, "Women doctors during the past 50 years have held a special place in the field of medicine." As an officer of the American Medical Association, the first woman to receive such an appointment, she was confident that women had helped to humanize the medical profession and "administered their scientific knowledge."

With a name like Slaughter, she might have eschewed surgery. She was born in 1876 in Lynchburg, Virginia. From the time her ancestors came from England to Virginia in the eighteenth century, seventeen of their direct and fifty-two of their collateral descendants became doctors. This heritage captured Rosalie's imagination. Her parents responded like the minister who, when calling on his congregation for volunteers to be missionaries, saw his own daughter rise and exclaimed, "Oh, my dear, I didn't mean you!"

In 1893 wealthy families expected a daughter to marry well and become a model mother. Rosalie's upbringing was not designed for a career. Her determination to be a doctor caused her family much anxiety.

Beatrice Bishop Berle in *A Life in Two Worlds* recorded a similar lifestyle before World War I: a girl in a well-bred family with old money was expected to travel to France, sometimes to attend school there, but especially to identify with the European aristocracy. Dr. Berle's parents decried her desire to go to Vassar and were appalled at her desire to study medicine.

Rosalie early on developed resourcefulness in a man's world. Her older brother John took her and another brother, Will, to the circus. Will exchanged three quarters for three tickets. When they came to the big tent, Will had only two tickets. In dismay, he said, "Rose, it's too bad. I lost your ticket."

"No, you didn't," responded little Rose, "You lost yours!" She gave him a hearty shove and walked in ahead of him. John murmured to the ticket man as he slipped him another quarter, "An emancipated woman."

Rosalie was twelve when the family sent her to Edge Hill, a private school directed by a descendant of Thomas Jefferson. At sixteen, applying to nursing schools, she met only rejection. She told her mother she really didn't want a lifetime of nursing. Relief showed in her mother's eyes until Rosalie added, "That would have been to get started. I really intend to be a doctor, like the boys." Rosalie's mother asked her why she did not want a comfortable life. The girl replied that Joan of Arc had become a soldier. Her mother exclaimed, "But she was burned at the stake!"

Her brother John offered encouragement from Duluth. If Rosalie became a doctor, he would welcome her to practice with him. By 1893 when Rosalie enrolled at Woman's Medical College in Philadelphia, successive classes of graduates had returned as faculty members. Two-thirds of the professors were women, among them Clara Marshall, from a prominent Quaker family who became dean of the college and professor of therapeutics. Marshall graduated from the college in 1875 and had been the first woman admitted to the Philadelphia College of Pharmacy, where she had taken honors. In 1882 she had taught obstetrics at the Philadelphia Hospital, the first woman on the staff.

Around the time Rosalie started medical school, nearly 130 women were serving on American hospital staffs.

Rosalie's enthusiasm for studying with a microscope and for pathology classes was due to her professor, Dr. Lydia Rabinovitch, who recently had been associated with the great German bacteriologist Dr. Koch in his discovery of the microorganism that caused tuberculosis.

Rosalie, after the death of her father, learned he had made no provisions in his will for his daughters, assuming they would marry and be supported by husbands. He provided for his wife and left the rest of his estate to his sons and grandchildren. She regarded her sudden financial independence as newfound freedom. In a severe Pennsylvania winter, she made a jacket of newspapers torn with a hole for her head. She claimed she carried a torch from hand to hand from the first American pioneer woman doctor, Margaret Jones, accused of witchcraft and the first person executed in Massachusetts Bay Colony. Joan of Arc was not her only heroine burned at the stake.

In the hospital, Rosalie would quote from the 1638 Connecticut blue laws about Jane Hawkins, the wife of Richard Hawkins, who was given three months to disappear or the "magistrates" would dispose of her. In the meantime she was forbidden to "meddle in surgery or phisick, drinks, plaisters, or oyles, nor to question matters of religion." Rosalie had only admiration for a Marlboro, Vermont, woman, Mrs. Thomas Whitemore, "possessed of a vigorous constitution and frequently travelling through the woods on snowshoes . . . to relieve the distressed."

During Rosalie's second medical school vacation, she worked ten hours a day in Massachusetts State Hospital, Tewkesbury, helping in the pharmacy, taking patient histories, recording physical examinations, and administering medicines. Slaughter's enthusiasm and professional interest endeared her to her patients, the paupers and discards of society. She offered them the sympathy they needed as much as medicine.

Before her final examinations, she delivered ten obstetrical cases, among them a poor woman who prayed her baby would not survive. Rosalie delivered a tiny infant, three and a half pounds, soon followed by a twin of the same weight. The poor mother cried, "Lord, take them back. I didn't want any more." She had despaired of caring for her six children, and now she had eight.

Rosalie Slaughter put her mouth to the infant's mouth to breathe life into the second baby. The young intern worked as hard at resuscitating the scrawny twins as she would the heirs to a fortune. The collapsed lungs gradually expanded, the spaces between the fragile ribs filled out, and the rhythm of breathing began.

Concluding the grueling obstetrical preparation for her medical degree, Slaughter filled an unexpired internship at Philadelphia City Hospital while studying at night for final examinations. Living in the hospital, she saved the costs of room and board. She wrote a full case history of pernicious anemia with lab reports and treatments in an essay that won the Alumnae Prize of $25 (which she spent on clothes).

On graduation day, just before Slaughter was to receive her degree of doctor of medicine, a telegram told her that her mother was dying. There was no train to Lynchburg for five hours; she received her degree in ice-cold hands and then took a train home. For a month she lovingly nursed her mother.

Dean Clara Marshall invited Slaughter to become resident physician of the Alumnae Hospital and Dispensary of the Woman's Medical College in Philadelphia. Dr. Slaughter worked there with five other women physicians from the college providing free care to the poor and ill.

Rosalie, primarily interested in gynecology, hoped to follow in the footsteps of her doctor brothers, who had studied in Vienna after graduating from the University of Virginia Medical School. "To be in the city of Mozart, Haydn, and Beethoven," Rosalie wrote, "to live in the most cosmopolitan place for education in the world—what a privilege."

Practicing frugality made it possible for her to work in the charity hospital in Vienna, then the largest in the world. Dr. Slaughter observed surgery and studied diagnosis in lung, heart, kidney, and other conditions. Rosalie was deeply disturbed by the unnecessary exposure of patients in the amphitheater when illness or surgery was demonstrated to classes. A poor woman in childbirth lay completely uncovered on a revolving table while students observed her agony for an hour and a half. Wealthy patients were handled with courtesy; the poor, with unfeeling harshness. Rosalie demanded an end to such humiliation.

In Vienna Dr. Slaughter met Samuel Clemens and his wife. The author expressed his admiration that Rosalie had become a physician.

In 1899 Dr. Slaughter, a lovely twenty-three-year old, accepted an invitation to spend Christmas in Russia. Among the men and women in fur coats and caps, she enjoyed an opera, Alexander Borodin's *Prince Igor*. She knew that the composer, a professor of organic chemistry, had been among the first to insist that women be allowed to study medicine. When the Medical School of Women was organized in 1878, Borodin played an incisive role in its founding.

From the opera, she was whisked back to her hotel, tucked into a horse-drawn troika, and luxuriously wrapped in rugs. She was asked to deliver some books to Leo Tolstoy, and the great man enjoyed her conversation so much, he invited her back repeatedly. "I have enjoyed talking to you as a comrade," he said. "We have crossed the thresholds of each other's minds."

Dr. Slaughter believed that diagnoses made by male doctors often were cruel to women. Men found it easy to dismiss a nervous woman as exaggerating her symptoms. She believed women actually suffered for years with an inflammatory or congestive condition, lacerations or tumors, neglecting to seek relief because of "modesty, poverty, or the mistaken idea that it is normal for women to have pain and endure it."

Later, in England, Slaughter studied in the laboratory of the celebrated brain surgeon Sir Victor Horsley. Helping with experiments on monkeys, she observed how pressure on various parts of the brain caused the monkey to move a finger, thumb, arm, or some other part of its body. After three years of postgraduate studies, she was pleased when Sir Victor offered her a permanent position. Did she want to do research instead of having her own practice? She was astonished at his next proposal. Would she consider returning to America by way of India?

The next thing she knew, she was spending six months in India treating patients with bubonic plague. She wavered constantly between fascination and horror. "Fakirs along the roadside, grotesque disfigurations, and self-imposed tortures."

In 1905 she met and married George Morton. Only a few years later, he died. She grieved for him and kept his name. Able to support herself, she avoided some of the indignities of other dependent widows. She taught medicine and had her own clinic with five assistants.

During the winter of 1915, her friends, Dr. Hans Zinsser of Columbia Medical and Dr. Richard Strong, returning from working to quell a typhus epidemic in Serbia, told Dr. Slaughter about conditions there. She sailed for

England in spring 1916, before America was drawn into the First World War. On the Salonica front in Greece, two English-speaking hospitals were operated by women: the American Unit of the Scottish Women's Hospitals in Macedonia and another on the Bay of Salonica. Dr. Slaughter wrote, "In our vast tent hospital and on the fields of Macedonia, we had 3,000 men under canvas, and never an empty cot."

Dr. Slaughter became a special commissioner of the Red Cross. She returned to the United States to help the American Women's Medical Association organize the War Service Committee, and in 1917 she took supplies to Serbia. The Medical Women's National Association arranged war service for women, and Rosalie designed the American Women's Hospital insignia.

After the war, Rosalie organized a program for Serbian students to pursue higher education in the United States. In addition to her private practice in New York, she was the first woman professor in the Medical School of Columbia University (1917–1918). In her autobiography, she described her desire to study social conditions in Iran, and by 1940 she published *A Doctor's Holiday in Iran* with her observations of clinics, missions, and women physicians in that troubled nation. In 1944 she presented a ten-foot statue of three heroic white limestone male figures, representing kindness, vision, and fortitude, to her birthplace, Lynchburg, Virginia.

Eventually, she moved to Winter Park, Florida, and continued private practice to a venerable age. She died in 1968 at age ninety-two.

Beatrice Bishop Berle

Beatrice Bishop's desire to be a doctor came much later in life than Rosalie's. Her parents opposed her independence, even forbidding her to go to Vassar. Thanks to a legacy from her grandmother, she was financially secure. She defied her deeply Francophile family, went to Vassar, and rejected her parents' opposition to Adolf Berle. When she and Adolf were married, neither of her parents came to the wedding. Beatrice and Adolf were married forty-three years and complemented each other with love and respect for each other's individuality.

After graduation from Vassar, Beatrice Bishop studied at the School of Social Work and became involved in fieldwork at the Bureau of Child Guidance. She relished contact with patients. Adolf encouraged her to join a summer staff in the small village of Pyne's Cove, Newfoundland, which had only ten houses. She taught school for the fishermen's children and considered her life goals. Now completely cut off from those goals, she became a psychiatric social worker in the Cornell Clinic at First Avenue. Later, she switched to teaching a course called History of the Family at the newly organized College of Sarah Lawrence in Bronxville.

In 1932 Adolf published *The Modern Corporation and Private Property.* Among his friends was Governor Franklin D. Roosevelt, who frequently invited the Berles to Hyde Park. In 1933 Adolf went to Cuba as financial advisor to the

American ambassador, and Beatrice registered at the College of Physicians and Surgeons of Columbia University, "buoyed," she wrote, "by Adolf's encouragement."

By 1938 Beatrice Bishop Berle received the longed-for medical degree from New York University and served briefly as an intern at Bellevue Hospital. When Adolf accepted an assignment with the State Department in 1939, they moved to Washington, and she did residencies at George Washington Medical School and Gallinger Hospital. Eventually, Dr. Thomas Parran, surgeon general of the United States Public Health Service, offered her a commission with the rank of major. Did Dr. Parran expect a married woman of forty with three children to organize an employee health service for government employees? Dr. Berle rejected the idea of becoming an administrator. At Gallinger Hospital she was studying tuberculosis and working with women in the diplomatic corps.

When the government sent the Berles to Brazil, Beatrice was eager to learn about that country's medicine. She applied to Santa Casa, a combination hospital and asylum for the aged or abandoned, a common institution in every Portuguese colony. Her fluent French was useful with the Sisters of Saint Vincent de Paul, many of them French, who were in charge of the twenty-bed wards. Besides doing rounds, Dr. Berle asked physicians to prepare lectures on public health problems in Brazil, and she herself wrote about the use of penicillin (a new subject in 1945).

On the family's return to New York, Dr. Berle became a fellow in medicine at the New York Hospital and Cornell University School of Medicine, where the clinic studied changes in color of exposed gastric mucosa, diabetes, peptic ulcers, asthma, and headaches.

During the 1950s, Adolf was involved in politics, international affairs, and establishing Le College de l'Europe Libre. His wife, in private practice, operated a clinic in East Harlem and published a book, *Eighty Puerto Rican Families: A Study of Health and Disease in Context*. The book evolved from a health facility in the East Harlem Protestant Parish that Beatrice ran with two colleagues, pediatrician Margaret Grossi and psychiatrist Marie Nyswander. This early experiment in community medicine was blessed by the arrival of Dr. Nyswander, who had experience in private practice treating heroin addicts.

Marie Nyswander

In 1979 marijuana was so available that even elementary school children smoked it. An Austin, Texas, policeman lectured at Doss Elementary School on the dangers of smoking pot. The next day a ten-year-old boy brought a marijuana plant for "show and tell." He said that the plants grew around the apartment complex where he lived.

New York City drug treatment clinics tested patients to determine the percentage of drug users infected with the AIDS (or acquired immune deficiency syndrome caused by a virus that attacks and destroys key elements in the immune system) virus and estimated that 60 percent of drug users in the city were infected in 1988.

At the same time, one in sixty-one New York City babies was born with antibodies to the AIDS virus. Similar catastrophes were reported in other American cities. Perhaps only half the New York babies with antibodies were actually infected with the AIDS virus; the others might eventually eliminate AIDS virus antibodies they acquired from their mothers. The infants would have to be fifteen months old before doctors knew if they actually carried the viral infection.

By the 1990s, AIDS had become an epidemic of worldwide concern. Federal grants to cities from the Center for Disease Control (CDC) in Atlanta provided testing and education for women at risk for the virus. The CDC recommended counseling and testing for women who had the AIDS infection, used intravenous drugs, were born in countries where heterosexual transmission of the disease was a major problem, or engaged in prostitution. The women were asked if they were sex partners of bisexual men, intravenous drug users, men with hemophilia, or men infected with AIDS.

What caused people, including children, from every walk of life to turn to drugs? The statistics became appalling, exacerbated by thousands of addicts returning from the Indochina War, and a widespread use of cocaine.

Dr. Marie Nyswander, a lithe woman who talked with her hands, became a heroine of storefront psychiatry and the war against drugs in New York. Good at creating and maintaining strong relationships with her patients, mostly East Harlem addicts, she impressed them because she had the courage to move into their neighborhood.

A young Puerto Rican addict confessed, "To talk real with any stranger is rough, especially when the stranger's a professional—you know, hey, better than you. Dr. Nyswander don't put us all in the same box. Other doctors use strange words and frighten us who ain't educated. I could blow my top for her. She blows her top too, believe me. If I light up a couple of cigarettes and just talk, she listens. Look, what it comes down to, I dig her. She swings. She's really alive."

Dr. Nyswander and her partner, Dr. Vincent Dole, were controversial figures in 1964 when they launched a program to use methadone to free heroin addicts from addiction. Methadone programs, costing an average of $1,500 a year for each addict, as opposed to $5,000 to $10,000 a year to imprison a convict, operated in most U.S. cities. Thousands of addicts clamored to enroll in these life-support programs. Methadone, when combined with psychiatric help, offered a highly motivated addict a chance to give up heroin. Developed as a morphine substitute in Germany during World War II, methadone relieved pain and eased the symptoms of heroin withdrawal without producing euphoria or the craving for ever-larger doses. Once hooked on heroin, methadone users might have had to continue indefinitely, as the heroin habit may alter the body's chemistry so crucially that life without opiates becomes impossible.

A sociologist on the staff of the East Harlem Protestant Parish Narcotics Committee, Seymour Fiddle, maintained, "The addicts made an art of guaranteeing their own failure." Of Nyswander he said, "Marie compelled these addicts to respond to her as total human beings. At first it was a shock for them to meet someone like her in a culture in which middle class people either avoid them or see them as part of an undifferentiated segment—the junky. They've been beaten by policemen, hounded by judges, betrayed by lawyers, wept over by social workers. Other psychiatrists working with addicts treat them only as addicts. Once you start treating them as human beings, they begin to feel they're human."

Why did Marie Nyswander specialize in addiction?

"I suppose the answer must include my reasons for being an analyst in the first place. I have a strong feeling for the beauty and dignity of man . . . I have a feeling for the joy experienced by others, or at least their capacity for joy, and their desire to be liberated from repression. I like to be in on the process of release if I can. That's what motivates me to treat addicts."

Writing about Dr. Nyswander, Nat Hentoff quoted her in *A Doctor among Addicts*: "In India and throughout the East, they've had their lotus eaters—their drug addicts—for centuries," she said. "They grow up with them, they feed them, and they consider the addict part of the whole community as a balance against the materialistic proclivities of their societies."

Dr. Nyswander claimed that addicts receiving legal methadone daily had no need to steal or murder. Crime in the cities may be largely due to heroin addicts trying to maintain expensive habits. Drugs contribute to a high suicide-attempt rate among heroin and cocaine addicts, perhaps fifteen times higher than that of non-addicts in the same age group. Treating addicts, Dr. Nyswander reflected, "requires a close look at their attitudes toward life and death and some respect for their depressions."

Nyswander revealed that 82 percent of the first 700 addicts who enrolled in her program in 1964 stayed with it: a remarkable success rate. Such results stem from social and economic aid, as well as from good medical care. For some of these addicts, the concern and compassion of the physician may have been the first care they had in their lives.

Heroin addiction was once concentrated in big American cities. In the 1990s, even affluent suburbs and Norman Rockwell hometowns had pushers and high school addicts who hungered for increasing amounts of drugs until the drug itself became the very object of life. Apathy and loss of appetite deplete the drug addict. Diseases such as pneumonia, tuberculosis, and VD were not the only threats as drug addiction became positively life-threatening. Addicts unable to study or hold a job began regarding themselves as worthless, and society reinforced this view.

To doctors involved in treating heroin addiction, methadone seemed a workable weapon, though it had drawbacks. It can be as addictive as the heroin it replaces. Doctors at the University of Chicago Pritzker School of Medicine experimented with a drug that is like methadone, 1-methadyl acetate, that suppressed withdrawal symptoms and narcotic hunger three times as long as ordinary methadone. The drug reduced temptations to cheat on treatment by selling heroin substitutes for money to buy drugs.

Dr. Nyswander, critical of the punitive approach to the addict, claimed that youth were attracted to drugs as an "adolescent way of rebelling and also of exploring life." At least a million sick citizens have been turned into criminals "virtually by a wave of the legislative wand," she said. In her campaign to turn the treatment of addicts over to doctors and do away with the stereotype of the addict, Dr. Nyswander wrote *The Drug Addict as a Patient* in 1956. More than forty years later, the United States continued to have the harshest laws and at the same time the worst narcotic problem of any country in the world—and the most complicated.

By 2000, though drug use in the United States had dropped, some of the nation's most prominent drug experts warned that the use of a psychedelic drug known as Ecstasy had risen sharply, particularly among youth. The U.S. Customs Service seized a record 8 million doses of Ecstasy at the nation's airports and other ports of entry in the months from October 1999 to August 2000. Officials believed these seizures represented a fraction of the Ecstasy that had been smuggled into the country. The drug increases energy and may foster a sense of well-being, and became popular with teens who gathered at nightclubs or held dance parties known as "raves." Drug traffickers with a pill costing 50 cents to manufacture sold one for up to $40.

Frances Oldham Kelsey

Although Dr. Helen Taussig was the first to warn of the dangers of thalidomide, Dr. Frances Kelsey became the eye of a storm that swept the Western world. Four years after thalidomide became available in Britain in 1958, some 4,000 deformed babies had been born. Doctors estimated that twice that number died at birth from internal injury. Promoted as a safe treatment for morning sickness and insomnia (though never sold commercially in the United States), thalidomide had been used experimentally in hospitals. In New York, reports of many deformed infants born in the same block led to a doctor who had sold "drug samples" to nearby pharmacists. They in turn resold them to pregnant women who came to them for medical care.

Dr. Taussig, learning of infants born with malformed limbs, some legless, armless, or earless, went to Europe to investigate these poor babies. Many had congenital heart problems; some had gastrointestinal malformations; some had kidney trouble; others were just cocoons of flesh with heads. Some of these infants became epileptic, some autistic, some mentally retarded. Taussig also determined that among the children who thrived, many had superior intelligence. Newspapers published pictures of babies with multiple malformations, fingers growing out of elbows, and disfigured faces.

Many parents were so deeply depressed they divorced or even committed suicide. Families lived in torment with thalidomide victims day by day. In Belgium, a crowd cheered when a couple was freed of murder charges in the poisoning of their legless eight-day-old baby.

In Germany where the drug was developed, more than $100 million in compensation was paid to thalidomide victims. The Distillers Company, the British licensee, a marketer of alcoholic beverages, was persuaded by consumer crusaders to increase dramatically the settlements to British, American, and Canadian victims on the threat of a possible boycott of their liquor.

In the United States, the American branch of Distillers Company had given some 2.5 million thalidomide tablets to doctors, who handed the drugs on to 20,000 patients. In 1962 *The Washington Post* implicated thalidomide in the birth of deformed infants and hailed Dr. Kelsey, then director of the Division of New Drugs of the U.S. Food and Drug Administration (FDA), for keeping the tranquilizer off the American market.

Dr. Kelsey, with a doctorate in pharmacology from the University of Chicago (1938), persisted in withholding approval of the drug. Worried about unproven side effects, she effectively blocked the sale of thalidomide in the United States despite the drug manufacturer's pressures on her.

Kelsey's predecessor in the FDA post, Dr. Barbara Moulton, resigned in 1960 in disgust, claiming harassment. Moulton, a well-qualified bacteriologist before becoming a physician, had studied antibiotics long before they became applicable to clinical medicine. As an assistant director of the Municipal Contagious Disease Hospital in Chicago, she had pursued research and taught antibiotic medicine. Dr. Moulton, familiar with foreign clinicians expressing shock over the obvious commercialism of the FDA program, came to realize that the emphasis of the program, instead of on consumer protection, was on approving drugs that the pharmaceutical industry wished to market. When she recognized that drugs indeed were approved before investigations were completed and that she could not change the situation, she resigned.

While serving in the FDA post, Dr. Kelsey considered the protection of the drug consumer her prime responsibility. She insisted on indisputable proof that thalidomide would be harmless to expectant mothers. As a result of her stubborn sense of duty, a fundamental human right was scrutinized: the right of patients to be free from taking medication without informed consent.

Working in a rickety Washington, D.C., barracks, Kelsey reasoned that the puzzling chemistry of thalidomide might cause paralysis of peripheral nerves. Two decades earlier, she had studied quinine's effects on rabbit fetuses. In the laboratory, she learned how drugs that irritate adult nerves could wreak havoc on the nervous controls of embryos. She observed stunted growth, malformations, and paralysis resulting from such drugs. Studying and experimenting with thalidomide, she saw that it had a harmful effect on animals. The poor beasts could not fall asleep. Examining and reexamining reports from England that the habitual use of the drug brought peripheral paralysis to some users, she was horrified but not surprised to learn about the unfortunate German babies.

Dr. Kelsey and her husband had two children. Her husband, pharmacologist Ellis Kelsey, following his wife's research, confirmed her reasoning. With his steady support she held fast to her refusal to approve the drug.

In 1962 President John F. Kennedy clasped about Dr. Kelsey's neck a ribbon dangling the Distinguished Federal Civilian Service Medal in honor of her heroic resistance to pressure and her consistent refusal to approve thalidomide for commercial sale. Thousands of American women joined the congratulations. Some of these women had never opened a science book in their lives, but they cared about what happened to luckless unborn babies. In 1970 when the longest trial in West Germany's history came to a close after two-and-a-half years of court sessions, newspapers reported that thalidomide had been responsible for the epidemic of malformed infants born between 1957 and 1961, affecting over 8,000 victims in forty-six countries.

In 1979, two decades after the thalidomide tragedy, Elaine Dale, who had been born without arms, gave birth to a healthy normal baby in Grimsby Maternity Hospital in England. Amidst tears of joy throughout the hospital, Dale cuddled her baby with her feet and said, "The sheer joy of having her makes up for all the pain in the world."

In 1996 researchers made an excruciatingly ironic announcement. They discovered what they believed are significant therapeutic uses for thalidomide, particularly against the complications of life-threatening ailments such as AIDS and cancer. The drug might be used against some AIDS-related conditions such as painful mouth ulcers and severe body wasting. Perhaps thalidomide would work in treating rheumatoid arthritis, glaucoma, lupus, or the chronic rejection state that can be deadly in bone marrow transplants. Thalidomide has been effective in treating leprosy in Mexico, the Philippines, South America, and Asia. Researchers hoped the drug could impact Crohn's disease, arthritis, multiple sclerosis, and Alzheimer's.

According to Dr. Debra Birnkrant of the FDA's division of antiviral drug products, "There is definitely a renewed interest in this drug, as long as it is controlled to ensure it is never given to pregnant women. It is definitely not a benign drug, but neither are the illnesses currently being treated with thalidomide in research. The goal is to get it only to patients who really need it."

Nancy Wexler

Nancy Wexler, a twenty-three-year-old psychologist when her mother was diagnosed in 1968 with Huntington's disease, promised herself she would devote the rest of her life to searching for the gene that causes this devastating illness.

Huntington's disease afflicted some 30,000 Americans in the last decade of the twentieth century. The inherited brain disorder inflicts disorientation, memory lapses, and deep depression. Patients die after a wretched decade or two of awareness of their decline.

In 1993 Nancy Wexler received the Albert Lasker Public Service Award, the highest honor in American medicine, for her groundbreaking work "toward finding a cure for Huntington's disease and for increasing awareness of all genetic disease." Though overwhelmed, she was quick to say, "We still do not have a cure."

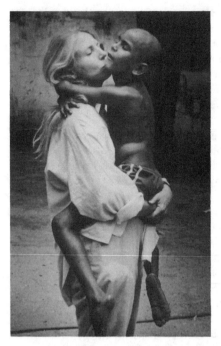

In 1972 Nancy Wexler learned of a population of Huntington's disease cases along the shores of Lake Maracaibo, Venezuela. Drawn to these people, she assembled a mission to the gene hunt. *(Photo courtesy of Nancy Wexler.)*

Nancy's mother, Leonore Wexler, a warm, nurturing parent, was a geneticist who studied fruit flies. When Nancy was in high school, she learned that all three of her mother's brothers had died from a relentless, fatal neurogenerative disease. Leonore had started college at fifteen, with a specialty in genetics. The only one of her family to go to a university, she had financial help from her two brothers, gifted musicians who played at the Tavern on the Green in New York City, and from a third, who was a salesman. In 1936 she was teaching high school in Harlem and dating a lawyer, Milton Wexler. Leonore encouraged him to leave law and earn a Ph.D. in clinical psychology. Leonore had been warned that no one would marry her if she revealed that her family had the disease, but she firmly believed that Huntington's affected only males.

In 1950 the family was devastated by the news that all three of Leonore's brothers, in their forties, had trouble with balance and memory problems. The brothers were diagnosed simultaneously with Huntington's.

On his sixtieth birthday, Milton Wexler invited his daughters, Nancy and her sister Alice, to dinner and informed them that Leonore also had Huntington's. He realized with regret that the behavior problems that had led to their divorce may have been symptoms of the fatal disease—silence, depression, irritability, and difficulty in relating to others. He promised his daughters he would support Leonore and care for her needs. Alice, then twenty-six, was well on her way to a doctorate in history at Indiana University. Nancy, having graduated from Radcliffe, had been accepted for graduate work in psychology at the University of Michigan.

Nancy proposed launching a research project immediately. "We may figure out a cure in time for mother." Within days of the diagnosis of Leonore's illness, Milton Wexler, "a tenacious guy" who had collaborated on several successful screenplays and had an active psychiatric practice, began devoting his life to establishing the Hereditary Disease Foundation that would fund the search for a cure.

Milton Wexler contacted Marjorie Guthrie, the widow of folk singer Woody Guthrie, the best-known victim of Huntington's chorea. The word "chorea" comes from the Greek for "dance," and for many years the common name was St. Vitus's dance. (Some of the women executed for witchcraft in colonial America may have been Huntington's victims.)

Marjorie Guthrie, organizer of the Committee to Combat Huntington's Chorea, urged Milton to form a California chapter to help lobby for research. Milton preferred to fund scientific research to lure dedicated researchers to workshops by paying for travel and brainstorming.

At one such workshop, Nancy learned about a research program using DNA markers that had never before been applied to hereditary disease where the chromosomal assignment of the gene was unknown. Nancy questioned: could research expand to large extended families with some sick and some healthy members?

While the Wexler family focused on finding a cure for Huntington's, Nancy kept her mother posted on every workshop, every grant funded, every new theory or proposed treatment, and every fund-raiser. In 1972 Nancy attended a symposium marking the hundredth anniversary of George Huntington's landmark paper that first described the disease. He had seen it as a boy, when he happened upon two tall, thin, cadaverous women who were bowing, twisting, and grimacing. By the time he became a doctor, he had observed three generations of sufferers and began to trace the hereditary pattern of the disease.

The symposium featured Ramon Avila Giron, a Venezuelan psychiatrist discussing a large population of related families all afflicted with Huntington's. They lived in villages around Lake Maracaibo in northwest Venezuela. Giron showed a grainy film with a tinny soundtrack. Nancy, astounded by the sight of people walking on the streets, sitting in outdoor cafes, dancing to the agony of the Huntington's gene, felt her heart quicken. Inbreeding, isolation, and large families (one man had thirty-four children) had produced a unique concentration of the mutant gene. These Huntington's victims, practically in every household, were not confined to nursing homes or stared at as they are in the United States, but accepted as part of a community.

Meanwhile Nancy and her sister pursued their careers. Nancy earned a doctoral degree in clinical psychology at the University of Michigan at Ann Arbor. She wrote her thesis on Huntington's disease and set up a Huntington's group in nearby Detroit to work with afflicted families.

In 1974, armed with her degree and glowing references, she looked for work. She worried that potential employers would become suspicious that she was at risk for Huntington's because of her obsession with it. With excellent credentials she was hired as a psychology teacher at the graduate level. Later she worked at the National Institutes of Health. When Congress mandated the Huntington's Disease Commission, Nancy became executive director. Her sister Alice, with a doctorate in history, wrote a biography of Emma Goldman and a book about Huntington's disease.

To help keep their mother from starving during her seven years in a nursing home, Nancy and Alice kept a small refrigerator in the room stocked with fattening food, cookies, and candy. At one sitting, Nancy wrote, her mother "polished off a pound of Turkish delight in half an hour with a grin of mischievous delight. She never gained weight; I gained weight eating to keep her company. I ate to keep from crying."

Nancy dressed her mother, bathed her, brushed her teeth, fed her, hugged and kissed her. Nancy and Alice decided they would never have children. Their beautiful, brilliant mother, like others who suffer from Huntington's disease, writhed and jerked in a bedroom chair, her fingers moving as if playing a piano, her legs and feet twitching constantly, sometimes working her way to the wall where she repeatedly hit the back of her head. Once an articulate scientist, Leonore Wexler had lost her ability to speak coherently. Until the end, on Mother's Day in 1978, Leonore always recognized her daughters.

Two years later, Nancy completed her doctoral thesis on the psychology of men and women at risk for Huntington's disease and went to New York to teach. However, her heart was already among the Maracaibo people, and she made two preliminary trips to Venezuela in 1979 and 1980.

In 1981 Nancy assembled ten volunteers to interview Venezuelan parents, grandparents, and children—the world's largest family (over 10,000 members) with Huntington's disease. The team collected blood and charted this extraordinary family tree. The lineage became the largest ever documented, more than 13,000 individuals. Nancy's group, sweating in the heat and swatting insects, explored barrios and worked in dispensaries or government-built clinics in outlying villages. Few people had ever had their blood drawn and they were frightened; some were suspicious and reluctant to cooperate. Wexler explained that the research might help find the cause of the disease, perhaps even a cure to benefit their children and grandchildren. Nancy told them that her mother had had the disease and that she and her sister were at risk. Possibly, in the distant past, she was related to them. The people seemed to bond to her; they responded.

Wexler's team discovered that all the Venezuelan victims descended from Maria Concepción Soto, who lived in the early nineteenth century. Wexler learned that the woman may have inherited the infection from her father, perhaps a European sailor, or by someone three generations before her. Nancy Wexler soon developed a genuine affection for the Huntington's disease victims. She grieved to see how the disease caused stiffening even in young people. Sitting at the bedside of a twenty-one-year-old Venezuelan woman who had been ill for five years, Wexler, in the habit of hugging, gathered the dying woman in her arms and received a slow radiant smile.

"I knew," Wexler said, "that locked in that woman's body was the answer to how Huntington's disease works."

A few years after Wexler's first trip to Venezuela, genetic researcher Jim Gusella and others discovered a marker for Huntington's disease, the first critical step toward finding the problem gene and developing treatments—even a possible cure.

Within a decade of research collaboration, an international group of six research teams from six institutions found the gene that causes Huntington's disease. This stunning first step stemmed from the Hereditary Disease Foundation created by Dr. Milton Wexler. Nancy praised the collaborators for generously sharing the results of their research.

Gusella's discovery also meant that the Wexler sisters, like anyone else, could determine if they had inherited the Huntington's gene. Milton, at eighty-five, felt that he did not want to end his life knowing his daughters were to have such a terrible finish to their lives. He objected to their taking the test, and neither woman would admit to having done so. Nancy strongly advocates keeping secret an individual's genetic makeup from employers, insurance companies, government, or any agency that might discriminate against people based on their genes. She and her sister realized that each had a 50 percent risk of inheriting the genetic disorder. In time, Nancy began to feel she had a huge family of thousands of people at risk for Huntington's around the world and that in her role at the center of the search for the gene, she would eventually help find a cure for all of them.

At the time the marker for Huntington's was discovered, Nancy met Dr. Herbert Pardes, head of the Columbia University Medical Center. His warm affection convinced her she could share the pleasures of life with him. They both knew enough about passing on the gene, and Nancy would neither have children nor burden him with a wife who had Huntington's. She and Dr. Pardes celebrated joy and contentment together. With her accomplishments, she felt personally and professionally fulfilled.

10

A Peaceful Revolution:
The Fight for Birth Control

The women have accomplished a peaceful revolution, and a beneficial one; and yet that has not convinced the average man that they are intelligent, and have courage and energy and perseverance and fortitude.

Mark Twain, *Following the Equator*, chapter 22

Use of contraceptives had been advocated in England as early as 1877 by Charles Bradlaugh and Annie Besant. They were hauled into court for selling Charles Knowlton's pamphlet *The Fruits of Philosophy* (subtitled *The Private Companion of Young Married People*). Written by a doctor, the book was for years the most important in the field and stressed Knowlton's response to the age-old charge that birth control was unnatural. "Sure it's unnatural," Knowlton agreed, "but so is cutting your fingernails or your hair. So is shaving. Civilization constantly wages war against nature."

The American Dr. Knowlton was tracked down in Massachusetts, arrested, tried, and sent to prison for three months at hard labor. Such a severe sentence was a bombshell in the medical community, striking the kind of fear in the hearts of doctors that the abortion issue aroused half a century later. However, in London, Dr. Knowlton's book was reprinted, complete with charts and illustrations. Bradlaugh and Besant brought out a third edition. This led to their arrest.

At her trial, Annie Besant declared she had counseled poor mothers who died young, worn out with too-frequent childbearing. Both Besant and Bradlaugh were sentenced to six months in jail.

"Family planning" was still a dirty phrase when two egocentric women claimed to have been the first to use the term "birth control." Both suffered incredible indignities in their struggles to disseminate information on family planning. "In a final estimate, Marie Stopes may well prove to have been one of the most important and outstanding influences of the twentieth century—a judgment with which, one feels sure, she would be in complete agreement," according to Margaret Pyke, chairman of the British Family Planning Association.

Of the American, Margaret Sanger, H. G. Wells wrote, "She's the greatest woman in the world." He predicted that within the century the birth control movement she launched would be so influential it would control human destiny.

Margaret Sanger

In 1914 when Margaret Sanger began her crusade, federal, state, and local laws were allied against her. She was jailed eight times according to her biographer, Emily Taft Douglas. Doctors denounced her. The clergy sermonized against her. Newspapers condemned her. Other reformers shunned her.

Marie Stopes's experiences of sexual and emotional unhappiness contributed to a career that she believed would put her in a "place with the immortals." Both Margaret Sanger and Marie Stopes were called "the Joan of Arc of family planning." If fanaticism makes a woman a Joan of Arc, these two crusaders qualify.

Margaret Sanger remembered how her spine froze at the sight of hundreds of poverty-stricken women lined up outside an abortion office waiting for the $5 curettement that might lead to mutilation, disease, and sometimes death. She had lost count of how many women she had seen "writhing in travail to bring forth babies." She was haunted by the sight of babies "wrapped in newspapers to keep them from cold; six-year-old children with pinched, pale, wrinkled faces . . . in gray, fetid cellars, crouching on stone floors, their small scrawny hands scuttling through rags . . . and white coffins, black coffins, coffins, coffins, interminably passing."

In her publication *Family Limitation*, Margaret Sanger wrote, "Every mother feels the wrong that the State imposes upon her when it deprives her of information to prevent bringing into the world children she cannot feed or clothe or care for."

Margaret Higgins was born in 1879 into a poor Catholic family in Corning, New York. As a teenager, she helped her father deliver her siblings, and became so confident and competent she delivered the neighbors' calves as well. At seventeen, she found school and home intolerable in Corning. She applied to and was accepted to a boarding school called Claverack College. She waited on tables to pay part of her tuition. She hoped to go to nursing school, but at twenty-two, she was in love with William Sanger, a twenty-nine-year-old architectural draftsman. His radical views impressed her. She wore an old blue dress when she and Bill eloped in 1902. In 1903 she gave birth to a nine-pound baby, Stuart. Margaret, like her mother, developed tuberculosis and lived in terror that the disease would kill her. Margaret's mother had had eleven children. Margaret was determined to limit the size of her family.

After her second son, Grant, was born in 1908, she presented a series of lectures on reproduction and sex, a first step in her lifelong career. A third child, Peggy, was born in 1911. The little girl was stricken with polio and died later of pneumonia, a loss that left a cloud over the family. Child care bored Sanger, and she paid as little attention as possible to her sons.

Sanger first attracted the attention of the press when 25,000 textile workers walked out on strike in Lawrence, Massachusetts, and 1,400 soldiers were rushed to the scene. Labor leaders were arrested. A trigger-happy soldier shot a young woman picketer. The strike might have ended then and there for parents needed to return to work when there was no food at home. The strikers, mostly Italian, adopted an Old Country practice and turned their children over for temporary adoption. A crusade of child care did not bore Sanger, a capable nurse, and she volunteered to chaperone the children to their temporary homes in New York. Before they left Lawrence, at her insistence a doctor examined the children and discovered one with diphtheria, several with chicken pox, and all of them undernourished, in thin rags against the bitter winter.

The press charged Sanger with staging a publicity stunt when journalists reported her role in the "Children's Exodus." Generous New York caretakers sent the youngsters home after six weeks, warmly dressed and in better health. As a result of the publicity, a socialist congressman, Victor Berger of Milwaukee, launched an investigation into conditions in the textile mills and called on Sanger to testify in Washington. In the crowded Rules Committee chamber, strikers' testimony was brushed aside as too emotional. However, Sanger's nursing experience helped her describe how malnourished and sick the children had been. Across the nation, newspapers carried Sanger's able testimony and a picture of the attractive young nurse.

In 1916 Margaret and her sister, Ethel Byrne, both professional nurses, opened a clinic in Brownsville, a Brooklyn slum. The police raided the clinic after only nine days, and both sisters went to prison for thirty days. Ethel Byrne was force-fed when she carried on a hunger strike.

The high mortality and unending misery Nurse Sanger observed among new mothers in tenements convinced her of the dire need for birth control. In 1921 Margaret Sanger organized the first American Birth Control Conference in New York City. Though she was still married to Bill, she carried on affairs with three other men.

That same year in November, what should have been Margaret's triumph, the opening of Malthusian League's clinic for poor mothers in South London, turned into a riot. The league had distributed thousands of leaflets. In a torrent of abuse, men, shouting "whores" and "abortionists," threw rotten eggs, stones, and apples at the staff and smashed in a door.

After World War II, Margaret Sanger decided to open a birth control clinic in London. She left her husband and children to see what she could learn from the British. Desolate and lonely in foggy London, she worked hard to get into the swim of opinion makers in England where birth control had become a burning issue. Marie Stopes wrote Sanger in 1920, "Mr. Roe and I have long planned to found our own birth control clinic in England as a memorial to our marriage."

Unlike Marie Stopes, who was an impressive speaker and relished performing before large audiences, Sanger preferred to address small groups. In

Scotland on the Fourth of July, Margaret Sanger declared her independence from excess children. At a socialist forum, she defied men who believed birth control would make poverty more tenable, bringing about reform that might retard the overthrow of capitalism.

"Well, then," countered Sanger, "why do you fight for higher wages? If misery is a weapon, why ask for an eight-hour day instead of a twelve- or fourteen-hour one?" She argued that women's rights were meaningless without some method of birth control.

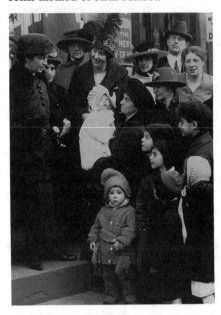

Margaret Sanger (far left) lectures on birth control to her enthusiastic clients. (*Photo courtesy of Planned Parenthood.*)

Near Andrew Carnegie's birthplace in Dunfermline, Sanger found poverty unchanged since the Industrial Revolution. Boys of eight or nine were apprenticed to the mines. Girls worked ten to twelve hours a day through their adolescence and up to the birth of their first child.

Sanger's plans to open a London clinic collapsed. Stopes opened what she claimed was the world's first birth control clinic on St. Patrick's Day—a day Marie may have chosen deliberately to defy the Catholic Church's campaigning consistently against her. The clinic was on Marlborough Road, Holloway, a slum area of North London in a house Marie and her husband, Humphrey, bought. For the first time in England, women could obtain free contraceptive advice.

In the meantime, Sanger, obsessed with the necessity of finding a cheap, acceptable contraceptive for the poor and uneducated, read about a chemical contraceptive in a German medical journal. She lost no time going to Germany to track down the chemist manufacturing the contraceptive jelly in Friedrichshaven. Though disappointed to find how expensive the jelly was, she bought a few samples. She interviewed German doctors, who were receptive until she explained her mission, and then they became angry. Germany needed babies to compensate for the men lost in the war.

"What about women who might die in pregnancy?" Sanger asked them. "Let the women have abortions."

"But abortions are illegal!" Should Germany allow mothers to determine the future of the master race? Such decisions must belong to doctors.

Saddened, Sanger returned to the United States. Before America entered the war, the New York Medical Society had strongly opposed birth control. By 1918 doctors had the right to prescribe contraceptives for a mother's health. Yet a survey of twenty-nine hospitals revealed that even women with tuberculosis or kidney problems were refused such help.

Sanger, hoping to open a birth control clinic staffed with doctors, wrote asking for support from many child specialists. The cynical replies reminded her that the more babies, the more business.

Margaret Sanger, who never went to college, was awarded an honorary doctorate in June 1949 from Smith College. To the end she believed that birth control would be "the cornerstone of that great structure: future civilization."

Marie Stopes

In England Margaret Sanger's leadership of the birth control movement was threatened by Dr. Marie Stopes, who had already opened her own clinic eight months earlier. Stopes's patients were being fitted with a small pessary inserted in the vagina. She had designed it herself and christened it a "Pro-Race" cap. She claimed responsibility for the creation of the birth control movement and regarded herself as its inventor. (However, rubber contraceptives that fitted over the neck of the uterus had originated in Holland, and French women had used them for decades.)

Marie Stopes, born in Edinburgh in 1880, was the daughter of J. F. Carmichael, a landscape painter, and Charlotte, the first woman in Scotland to take a university certificate—the only qualification open to women even if they had succeeded in examinations. This denial, and the fact that women were not allowed to attend lectures or be awarded degrees, made Charlotte, a Shakespearean scholar, an advocate of women's suffrage all her life. Surprisingly she always openly envied her daughter's scholarly successes.

By the time Marie enrolled in the science faculty of a woman's college attached to London University, women could take degrees. Though she wanted to take honors in chemistry, her strongest subject, she was refused. When a professor of botany agreed to allow her to take honors, she attended both evening and daytime courses. At the end of the year, she won a gold medal in botany. When her dearly beloved father developed cancer, Marie offered evidence of her devotion and achievements by earning her degree and taking double honors in two years. She received the university's Gilchrist Scholarship, entitling her to a year's postgraduate work abroad. In 1903, not yet twenty-three, Marie took a boat train to Munich, intending to dedicate her life to science and to the study of the reproductive aspects of early plant life.

No woman had ever been allowed to take a university doctorate from the Botanical Institute in Germany. Marie persisted, working twelve hours a day. In the end, university regulations were changed, allowing her to present her thesis on the cycads and defend it in German. She was now Dr. Marie Stopes, the first woman ever to earn a doctorate in botany in Germany.

In the laboratory, she had met a thirty-seven-year-old Japanese student, Kenjiro Fujii. Neither wanted to admit a physical attraction. A few years later Fujii visited her briefly in Manchester. Marie was working for her London doctor of science degree, which she took in 1905. She became the youngest doctor of science in Britain, collaborating with Fujii on botanical research. In Manchester, Marie studied coal, insisting on going down into the mines herself rather than having samples brought to her.

With the idea of a trip to Japan reinforcing her scientific curiosity, Marie applied to the Royal Society for a grant to go to Japan in the summer of 1907. During her eighteen months there, her love affair with Fujii withered.

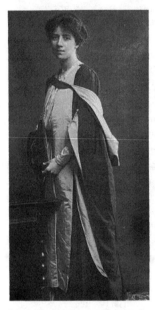

Marie Stopes became famous for her book *Married Love*. *(Photo courtesy of Harcourt, Brace, and Jovanovich.)*

Back in England, Marie accepted the first man who proposed to her. She was so sexually naive that she was married six months before she realized her husband was impotent. Now thirty-seven, overcoming a failed love affair and an annulled marriage, she met Humphrey Roe, young, handsome, and wealthy. They were married, and he joined her efforts to promote birth control.

She was amazed to discover that sex could be exciting. She wrote *Married Love* and submitted the manuscript to a number of publishers, among them Stanley Unwin, who wanted to publish it. His colleague disagreed. Blackie & Son had published her *Ancient Plants* and letters she had received from Fujii, *A Journal from Japan*. The letters were obviously an invasion of Fujii's privacy even though they were slightly fictionalized. Walter Blackie wrote her: "Dear Dr. Stopes, Thanks. But the theme doesn't please me."

Marie was considering publishing it herself when she met Margaret Sanger and asked her to circulate the manuscript in America. *Married Love* was published and became an instant success. In England, a minor publishing house, A. C. Fifield, accepted it in 1918. In both countries, more than a million copies were sold. Marie Stopes was famous.

When Stopes claimed that her birth control clinic was the first in the English-speaking world, Margaret was so furious that forever after, the two women were enemies.

The Catholic Church bitterly opposed both Margaret Sanger and Marie Stopes. Sanger wrote about impoverished mothers spending their last dollar to bury a baby with a Mass. For years afterward, they paid out precious pennies for candles in remembrance of the dead child.

Neither Margaret Sanger nor Marie Stopes seemed able to have serene, satisfactory relationships with lovers or husbands, yet these two crusaders did more for birth control than any other women of the twentieth century.

11

What Was the Doctor Wearing?: From White Coats to Space Suits

How poor they are that have not patience!
What wound did ever heal but by degrees!
Shakespeare, *Othello*, Act I, Scene 3

In 1881 a South Carolina student at Harvard Annex (the school that was a precursor of Radcliffe) became ill and was attended by a woman doctor. Reporting this remarkable event, author Carol Bleser in *The Hammonds of Redcliffe* said that not a word was recorded about the treatment or medication or results of the woman physician's ministrations. What we get instead is a minute description of what the doctor was wearing!

We know that when Dr. Mary Walker wore pants during the Civil War, she was not only criticized, she was ridiculed and harassed. In the twenty-first century, from muumuu to space suit, nothing surprises us. The white coat has long been a uniform for medical professionals, and no one is surprised that brand new medical students at Columbia University's College of Physicians and Surgeons (and elsewhere) don white coats and recite the Hippocratic oath at initiation ceremonies welcoming them into the medical community. An associate dean of student affairs, Dr. Lina Lewis, called the coats "cloaks of compassion—symbols of the value of humility in their careers."

Dorothy Brown

Founded in 1876 in Nashville, Tennessee, Meharry Medical College is the largest private historically black college dedicated to educating health care professionals and biomedical students in the United States. With a heritage of caring for the health of the disadvantaged of all origins, Meharry College had

189

graduated more than 3,000 African-American physicians by 2001. Originally women were educated only as nurses and midwives.

Several African-American women who aspired to be doctors were eventually awarded degrees from the Woman's Medical College of Pennsylvania. They became guardians of the health of black women. Among these notable doctors were Rebecca J. Cole (1867), Lulu (Louise) Fleming (1895), Eliza Anna Grier (1897), Matilda Arabell Evans (1897), and Virginia Margaret Alexander (1925).

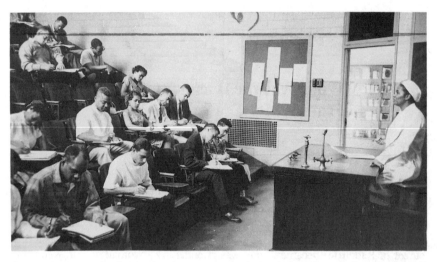

Dr. Dorothy Brown, the first black woman surgeon in the South, lecturing a medical class in 1958 wearing a white coat. *(Photo courtesy of Meharry Medical College.)*

Sarah Elizabeth Pierce-Emerson

What did the Hawaiian doctor Sarah Elizabeth Pierce-Emerson wear? In the nineteenth century, she probably turned to the long graceful muumuu that makes Hawaiian women look so lovely.

In the annals of women medical doctors, few made a greater contribution in pioneering to break the barriers to higher education for women than Sarah Emerson, who gave up a successful New York practice to respond to the request of the Hawaiian Board of Health to work in Honolulu.

She was born in Fall River, Massachusetts, in 1855, the second daughter of Captain Abraham Wilcox Pierce and Harriet (Durfee) Pierce. Sarah's father, a whaling captain who sailed from New Bedford for the Pacific and Honolulu with his family on board, took Sarah on her first voyage before she was two years old. When Sarah was four years old, Captain Pierce arrived in Honolulu Harbor for the ninth time.

That year the Pierces found the balmy breezes of Honolulu so appealing that they bought a house in Oahu. But for economic reasons, the family returned to New Bedford where Captain Pierce opened a store for shippers.

The family came home to Honolulu when Sarah was eighteen. Her father believed that medical secrets lurked in the botanical gold mine of rain forests. His fascination with Hawaiian herbal medicines shaped Sarah's desire to be a doctor. She was accepted by Boston Medical School in 1872. When she walked into class, male students and some professors objected so vocally that Sarah withdrew after two weeks.*

She promptly enrolled at Boston University in liberal arts. A brilliant student, she later convinced Boston Medical School to allow her to reenroll. To pay her tuition she tutored other students. She earned her M.D. degree in 1875.

Now a doctor, she wanted to further her medical training as other women doctors of her era did by studying in Europe. In hospitals of Leipzig, Dresden, and Paris, she saw new treatments in pediatrics and gynecology.

Back in America in 1878, she met Dr. N. B. Emerson in New York, who became a warm friend. He was a son of missionaries in Hawaii. Sarah's practice was confined to treating women and children. In 1882 she returned to Honolulu with her older sister, Harriet.

Licensed by the kingdom's Board of Health in 1883, Sarah Pierce was one of the first of two women doctors at the time in Hawaii. The other was Dr. Frances M. Wetmore. When N. B. Emerson returned to Hawaii, he called on Sarah, and their mutual respect blossomed into love. They were married in 1885. Dr. Pierce practiced medicine until the birth of her only child, Arthur Emerson, in 1887. After that she devoted less time to her medical practice and more to her enthusiasm for Hawaiiana. She tutored students in French, German, and Latin. The Emersons, magnetized by Hawaiian culture and history, made lasting contributions to the state. Dr. Pierce died in 1938 in Honolulu.

*University of Hawaii library resources.

Ruth Kleinfeld Lenney

At the University of Hawaii Medical School, Dr. Ruth Kleinfeld Lenney, who sometimes teaches in a muumuu, observed that medical school classes from now on may be 50 percent women. "Their influence creates a gentler environment. Many of the students who come in now are motivated by dedication to medicine. They share a sense of compassion and caring. In tutorials, it is usually women who worry about the influence of a patient's illness on the family. Of course, I sometimes have an insensitive female student. When women are in internships, they may come up against men who were educated in the old system. We hope that students will be challenged by sensitive physicians, particularly in psychiatry, who teach the importance of compassion in medicine."

Lenney said that women psychiatrists in practice often treat "fashionable ladies" who confess they are tired of shopping and "trying on." The patient may protest she is not interested in a profession but is discontented. The sympathetic psychiatrist may help the woman deal with the truth. What a woman wears is not her whole life.

Statistics reveal that in the last decades of the twentieth century, troubled women who experienced an "empty couch syndrome" began seeking a female therapist in an attempt to remove themselves from the traditional "man in power–woman subservient" model. This trend accelerated with reports that patients had been sexually harassed or even raped by a male therapist. Nancy A. Roeske, professor of the Department of Psychiatry, Indiana University School of Medicine, contended that women's personality characteristics—intuitive, patient, verbally skillful, empathetic—are particularly suitable for the role of psychiatrist.

Rhea Seddon

In 1983 Sally K. Ride was the first U.S. woman astronaut to go into space. Two other medical doctors, Rhea Seddon and Ann Fisher, were involved early on in the American space program. Wendy Lawrence, daughter of a test pilot who trained with the first astronauts, had helicopter flight training after earning a master's degree in oceanography from MIT. Though not an M.D., Lawrence joined the astronaut corps in 1992 and was among those (including Dr. Rhea Seddon) who finished an orbital repair job on the Hubbell Space Telescope in December 1993.

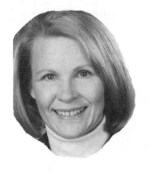

Rhea Seddon met her husband, Professor Marshall Fishwick, in the astronaut corps, and they have three children. After graduating from the University of Tennessee College of Medicine in 1973, Seddon completed a surgical internship and three years of a surgery residency in Memphis. Her special interest was surgical nutrition. In Houston, Texas, she combined her work as an astronaut with serving in hospital emergency rooms. Chosen as a candidate by NASA in 1978, Seddon became an astronaut in 1979. She made her first space journey on the fourth flight of Discovery and the sixteenth shuttle mission from Kennedy Space Center in Florida in 1985. During the nine-day mission, she helped perform experiments in exploring how humans, animals, and cells respond to microgravity and readapt to Earth's gravity on return. She was payload commander of the Spacelab Life Sciences mission in 1993.

Dr. Rhea Seddon was chosen as an astronaut in 1979. (*Photo courtesy of NASA.*)

Patricia A. Santy

What does the woman astronaut wear in space? The question needed serious consideration, and it fell to Dr. Patricia Santy to engage in research on the psychophysiological aspects of space travel. She examined the height and reach differences of men and women that influenced the design and instrumentation of equipment on board a spacecraft.

"In our lifetime," she wrote, "we will probably see the beginnings of the colonization of space. I have no doubt that such colonization will mark the most important series of events in the history of mankind. As a psychiatrist as well as a scientist, I believe that the ultimate success or failure of this great human endeavor will hinge considerably on many psychiatric factors."

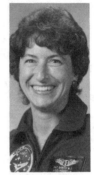

Patricia Santy, psychiatrist, teacher, and scientist. *(Photo courtesy of NASA.)*

Patricia Santy, born in 1949, earned a master's degree in biomedical engineering at Marquette University, Wisconsin; a second master's in biological chemistry; and an M.D. at UCLA Harbor Medical Center, Torrance, California, where she won the "Outstanding Teacher Award" in 1981.

Writing about what women in space wore, she said, "If women are to be part of the crew, then the spacecraft must be designed so that people of all heights and reaches are able to operate the machines."

Space suits were designed for men, their weight and size obviously unsuitable for women. "Garments need to be tailored specifically for women," Santy insisted. "Waste collection in the space suit as designed for men—a tube around the penis—is obviously inadequate for women. The 'Disposable Absorption Containment Trunk,' a combination diaper and long-line panty girdle, was designed."

Hair length was an issue, since long hair in zero gravity can be a nuisance. Santy recommended that personal groom kits issued to women include cosmetics and something to help the women manage menses in flight. No one could predict how effective tampons or other internal collection methods would be in zero gravity.

Two hundred women pilots were subjected to tests of urinary stress incontinence and induced menstrual flow, weightlessness tolerance, and G tolerance. G stress is that dreaded force that pins a pilot against the seat as the craft throttles up to full speed and accelerates into the sky or out of the Earth's atmosphere. Women pilots showed a tolerance for coping with G forces comparable to that of men, and their tolerance seemed significantly higher during menstruation.

Shannon Lucid

On March 22, 1996, U.S. astronaut Shannon Lucid began what was expected to be a four-and-a-half-month journey to live and work aboard the ten-year-old Russian Mir space station. Lucid, a fifty-three-year-old biologist and mother of three grown children, was the first woman to hold a major American space-flight record for which either gender was eligible.

Before blasting off on the American shuttle to be a guest on the Russian space station, she studied the Russian language. Lucid's stay in space was extended to six months when shuttle booster problems and two hurricane threats delayed the launch of Atlantis, which was to bring her back to Earth. Her voyage ended after 188 days on September 26, 1996, as the shuttle Atlantis landed at NASA's Kennedy Space Center in Florida.

Her flight established not only a new U.S. space flight endurance record but also a new world's record for the longest mission by a woman. Lucid was the first woman ever to be awarded the Congressional Space Medal of Honor. In an Oval Office ceremony on December 1, 1996, President Bill Clinton called her "our American hero, Shannon Lucid" and praised her as a "determined vision-ary, a pioneer whose example inspires young Americans."

During her months in space, she maintained her natural good spirits, though she missed her family and friends, bookstores, M&M candies and potato chips, and a good hot shower.

Shannon Lucid, born in 1943 in Shanghai, was the first child of Oscar and Myrtle Wells, U.S. missionaries in China. Her mother's childhood was spent in China with her father, whose Dutch church had sent him as its first missionary to the Orient.

Shannon was an infant when the Chinese incarcerated the family with forty-seven other British and American prisoners. For two years they all crowded into two bedrooms of an old university. The Wellses left China for India on a ship crowded with over 1,500 refugees. To avoid mined waters, the ship circumnavi-gated the world, a voyage lasting seventy-six days.

After World War II the family returned to China as missionaries. Shannon learned to like strange Chinese food and riding rickety buses. When she was eight, she flew from Shanghai across the Kuling Mountains in an antique, unpressurized airplane. Shannon observed that the pilot was "just a human being and I decided right then and there when I grew up I would learn how to fly."

The family left China again when the communists gained control of the country. Shannon, in high school in Oklahoma, wrote an essay about her dream of becoming a rocket scientist and flying in space. An unusually fine student, she used the term "astronaut" before it ever made headlines. Her teacher would not accept the essay because Shannon "had not cited sources."

For her school's science fair, she needed a teacher's permission to buy chemicals for an experiment on inhibitory factors that might prevent cancer in mice. This request was granted but not with enthusiasm. Shannon won first place and later took top prize in the regional competition. Even after she received the Bausch and Lomb Science Award and had graduated in 1960 with "high honor," one of her teachers warned her about her plans to go to college. "Why waste your parents' money?"

Undaunted, Shannon enrolled at the University of Oklahoma and earned bachelor's, master's, and doctorate degrees in science.

When she married Michael Lucid, he promised to support her aspirations to become an astronaut, even if they had to move to Texas. The Lucids had three children: Kauai Dawn in 1968; Shandara Michelle, 1970; and Michael, 1975.

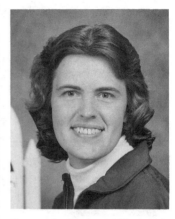

In 1978 Shannon was among the first group of women candidates selected for NASA's astronaut training. In 1979 she completed training as a mission specialist on space shuttle flight crews. In 1985 she made her first flight on an eight-day mission that included satellite deployments and X-ray astronomy experiments. By 1996 she had had five career space flights, the most of any woman in the world. "I love looking out the windows from the flight deck when I have time off." She sacrificed sleep to gaze out the window at that awesome small globe floating in space where every ninety minutes, another sunrise and a sunset looks over the rim of the world.

Shannon Lucid spent 188 days in space. *(Photo courtesy of NASA.)*

The Russian Space Agency publicly praised Lucid for her "patience." Lucid reported that every time they left Mir for a space walk, her Russian colleagues told her, "You're in charge but don't touch the controls."

Two weeks after her return to Earth from this record-setting event, Lucid said she would be willing to go up on the next shuttle flight, "but don't tell my husband."

Eileen Collins

Following the triumphs of Sally Ride, the first U.S. woman in space, and of Shannon Lucid, the announcement in 1998 that a woman would command a NASA space shuttle was no longer amazing. Amid pomp and ceremony during a week of emphasis on space and science at the White House, First Lady Hillary Rodham Clinton announced that Air Force Lt. Col. Eileen Collins would be the first woman to command a NASA space shuttle.

Collins, forty-one, had already clocked over 400 hours in space. In 1995 she became the first woman to pilot a space shuttle, sitting at the controls for the first flight of the Russian-American Space Program, a joint venture featuring a rendezvous with the space station Mir.

Collins was also the pilot on a 1997 mission that included a docking with Mir. Her shuttle mission would include carrying an X-ray telescope into space.

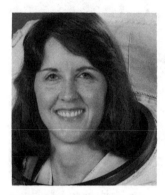

Collins had already served twice as a shuttle pilot for missions in 1995 and 1997 and was therefore in line for the position of shuttle commander.

She became an astronaut in 1991. The mother of one child, Collins, a New Yorker, was married to Pat Youngs in San Antonio, Texas.

Kathryn C. Thornton

So many women made commitments to opening the frontier of space that their courage may sometimes seem commonplace. Dr. Kathryn C. Thornton earned a Ph.D. in physics at the University of Virginia in 1979. With two stepsons and three daughters, she served on the crew of the maiden flight of the space shuttle *Endeavor*. During the mission the crew conducted the initial test flight of Endeavor and performed four space walks to demonstrate and evaluate tests needed to assemble the Space Station Freedom. Later, Thornton was among the group that was called "Dr. Goodwrenches" in the repair mission of the Hubble Space Telescope. She perched on top of the shuttle's fifty-foot arm and sent a mangled solar-energy panel into space, as *Time*

Dr. Kathryn Thornton was a crew member on Endeavor. *(Photo courtesy of NASA.)*

reported in the December 20, 1993, issue, "like a falconer letting her bird take wing." She shouted, "Piece of cake."

Bibliography

Ackerman, Jennifer, "Journey to the Center of the Egg — Nobel Prize Winner C. Nusslein-Volhard," *New York Times Magazine* (May 1994): 42–45.

Addams, Jane, *Twenty Years at Hull-House* (New York: Macmillan, 1929).

Alsop, Gulielma Fell, *History of the Woman's Medical College* (Philadelphia: Lippincott, 1950).

Anderson, Louisa Garrett, *Elizabeth Garrett Anderson (1836–1917)* (London: Faber and Faber, 1939).

Baker, Nina Brown, *Cyclone in Calico* (Boston: Little, Brown and Company, 1952).

Barringer, Emily Dunning, *Bower to Bellevue: The Story of the First New York Woman Ambulance Driver* (New York: Norton, 1950).

Bell, Enid M., *Storming the Citadel: The Rise of the Woman Doctor* (London: Constable, 1953).

Berle, Beatrice Bishop, *A Life in Two Worlds* (New York: Walker Co., 1983).

Blackwell, Elizabeth, *A Curious Herbal* (London: John Nourse, 1837).

———, *Medicine as a Profession for Women* (New York: W. H. Tinson, 1860).

———, *Pioneer Work in Opening the Medical Profession to Women* (New York: Longmans Green, 1895).

Blake, John B., "Women and Medicine in Anti-Bellum America," *Bulletin of the History of Medicine* 39, no. 2 (1965): 99–123.

Bluemel, Elinor, *Florence Sabin, Colorado Woman of the Century* (Boulder: University of Colorado Press, 1959).

Bollinger, Edward Taylor, *Rails That Climb—The Story of the Moffat Road* (Santa Fe: Rydal Press, 1950).

Branch, Patricia, *Silent Sisterhood: Middle Class Women in the Victorian Home* (London: Croom Helm, 1975).

Carreau, Mark, "Lucid Thinks About a Repeat," *Houston Chronicle,* 11 October 1996, 8A.

———, "Lucid Welcomes Colleagues to Mir," *Houston Chronicle,* 20 September 1996, 11A.

Chang, Ina, *A Separate Battle: Women and the Civil War* (New York: Dutton, 1991).

Chase, Julia A., *Mary A. Bickerdyke, "Mother"* (Lawrence, Kan: Journal Publishing House, 1896).

Cimons, Marlene, "It's All in the Family," *Los Angeles Times Magazine*, 10 February 1991, 8–12.

Clarissa Harlow Barton Papers, Manuscript Department, Duke University Library, Durham, N.C.

Cohen, Elisabeth, *Rachel Forster Hospital: The First Fifty Years* (Sydney, New South Wales: Rachel Forster Hospital, 1969).

Colvin, Michael, "Gertrude Belle Elion (1918–1999)," *Science* (28 May 1999).

Commager, Henry Steel, *The Blue and the Gray* (New York: Fairfax Press, reprint 1982), 412–13.

Cope, Zachary, *Florence Nightingale and the Doctors* (New York: Museum Press, 1958).

Curie, Eve, *Madam Curie,* translated by Vincent Sheean (New York: Doubleday, 1938).

Dally, Ann Cicely, *The Story of a Doctor* (London: Gollancz, 1968).

Davis, Margaret Burton, *Mother Bickerdyke and the Soldiers* (San Francisco: A. T. Dewey, 1886).

Dengel, Anna, "The Work of Medical Women in India," *Medical Woman's Journal* 37, no. 5 (1930): 132–35.

———, "The Work of the Medical Mission Sisters in India," *Medical Woman's Journal* 49, no. 9 (1942): 263–67.

Dowell, William, "The Sand Fly Saga: Jill Seaman and Kala-Aza," *Time* (Special Issue) 150, no. 19 (1997): 80–81.

"Down to Earth," *Newsweek* (7 October 1996): 31–36.

Dreifus, Claudia, "Joyce Elders," *The New York Times Magazine* (30 January 1994).

Dugger, Celia W., "Modern Asia's Anomaly: The Girls Who Don't Get Born," *The New York Times,* 6 May 2001, "Week in Review," 4.

Edmonds, Emma, *Nurse and Spy in the Union Army* (Hartford, Conn.: W. S. Williams & Company, 1895).

Evans, Sara M., *Born for Liberty: A History of Women in America* (New York: The Free Press, 1989).

Fraser, Antonia, *The Weaker Vessel* (New York: Alfred A. Knopf, 1984).

Gollaher, David, *Voice for the Mad: The Life of Dorothea Dix* (New York: The Free Press, 1995).

Goodfield, June, *An Imagined World: A Story of Scientific Discovery* (New York: Harper & Row, 1981).

Gray, Madeline, *Margaret Sanger: A Biography of the Champion of Birth Control* (New York: Richard Marek, 1979).

Guttentag, M., and H. Bray, *Undoing Sex Stereotypes* (New York: McGraw Hill, 1976).

Hacker, Carlotta, *The Indominable Lady Doctors* (Toronto: Clarke, Irwin & Co., 1974).

Hall, Ruth, *Passionate Crusader: The Life of Marie Stopes* (New York: Harcourt, Brace & Jovanovich, 1977).

Hamilton, Alice, *Exploring the Dangerous Trades* (New York: Little, Brown and Co., 1943).

Hemenway, Ruth V., *M.D. Medical Woman's Journal* 52, no. 2 (1945).

Hentoff, Nat, *A Doctor among the Addicts* (New York: Rand McNally, 1968).

Holland, Mary A. Gardner, *Our Army Nurses* (Boston: B. Wilkins & Company, 1895).

Horney, Karen, *New Ways of Psychoanalysis* (New York: W. W. Norton and Co., Inc., 1950).

Hume, Ruth Fox, *Great Women in Medicine* (New York: Random House, 1964).

"Huntington's Gene, So Near, Yet So Far," *Science* (February): 624–25.

Keller, Evelyn Fox, *A Feeling for the Organism: The Life and Work of Barbara McClintock* (San Francisco: W. H. Freeman & Co., 1983).

Kellogg, Florence S., *Mother Bickerdyke as I Knew Her* (Chicago: Utility Publishing Co., 1907).

Kerner, Charlotte, *Lise, Atomphysikerin: Die Lebensgeschichte der Lise Meitner* (Berlin: Beltz & Gelbert, 1989).

Levin, Beatrice, *Women and Medicine, 2d ed.* (Lincoln, Neb.: Media Publishing, 1989).

Lewis, Loyd, *Sherman, Fighting Prophet* (New York: Harcourt, Brace and Co., 1932), 362–65.

Lovejoy, E. P., *Women Doctors of the World* (New York: Macmillan, 1957).

Mary Norton Papers, 1852–1895, Manuscript Department, Duke University Library, Durham, N.C.

McGrayne, Sharon Bertsch, *Nobel Prize Women in Science* (Secancus, N.J.: Carol Publishing, 1993).

Miller, Susan Katz, "To Catch a Killer Gene," *New Scientist* (24 April 1993), 37–41.

"Mrs. Elgood," *Medical Woman's Journal* 30, no. 10, (October 1923): 309–10.

Nyswander, Marie, *The Drug Addict as a Patient* (New York: Gruen and Rowe, 1956).

O'Malley, Ida Beatrice, *Florence Nightingale 1820–1856* (London: Thornton, 1931).

Opfell, Olga S., *The Lady Laureat: Women Who Have Won the Nobel Prize, 2d ed.* (Metuchen, N.J.: Scarecrow Press, 1986).

Phillips, B., "Mary Walker, First Woman Doctor in the Army," *The New York Times Magazine* (11 July 1943): 28.

Putnam, Ruth, ed., *Life and Letters of Mary Putnam Jacobi* (New York: Putnam, 1915).

Randall, Fredericka, "The Heart and Mind of a Genius," *Vogue* (March 1987).

Revkin, Andrew, "Hunting Down Huntington's," *Discover* (December 1993) 98–108.

Robinson, Marion O., *Give My Heart: The Dr. Marion Hilliard Story* (New York: Doubleday & Co., 1964).

Ross, Ishbel, *Child of Destiny* (New York: Harper & Row, 1949).

Rossi, B., "Florence Sabin," *The Johns Hopkins Journal* 7 (1959), 7-12.

Rubin, Jack L., *Karen Horney, Gentle Rebel of Psychoanalysis* (New York: Dial, 1978).

Sanger, Margaret, *An Autobiography* (New York: Norton, 1938).

Sciolino, Elaine, "The Chanel under the Chador," *The New York Times Magazine* (4 May 1997): 46–51.

Seidenberg, R., "Images of Health, Illness and Women in Drug Advertising," *Journal of Drug Issues* 4 (1967): 264–67.

Siebel, Johanna, *The Life of Dr. Marie Heim Vogtlin, the First Swiss Woman Physician* (Zurich, Switzerland: Rashcer & Co., 1919).

Smith, Elizabeth, *A Woman with a Purpose: The Diaries of Elizabeth Smith (1871–1884),* ed. Veronica Strong-Boag (Toronto: University of Toronto Press, 1980).

Smith, Roy G., "Behind the Veil in Saudi Arabia," *Pacific Health* 12 (1979): 2–5 (published by the School of Public Health, University of Hawaii, Honolulu, Hawaii).

Snyder, Charles McCool, *Dr. Mary Walker: The Little Lady in Pants* (New York: Vantage Press, 1964).

Sonnenborn, Liz, *Clara Barton, Founder, American Red Cross* (New York: Chelsea House Publishers, Main Line Book Co., 1992).

Steinmann, Marion, "Nancy Wexler's Quest for a Cure," *Columbia* (November 1987): 15–19.

Svartz, Nanna, *Step by Step: An Autobiography* (Stockholm, Sweden: Albert Bonniers, 1968).

Tabor, Margaret E., *Elizabeth Blackwell: The First Medical Woman* (London: The Sheldon Press, 1925).

Van Dyke, Robert, *Notable Women of Hawaii,* ed. B. B. Peterson (Honolulu: University of Hawaii Press, 1984), 115 ff.

Wexler, Nancy, "Life in the Lab," *Los Angeles Times Magazine* (10 February 1991), 12 ff.

White, Ron, "Shannon Lucid, Astronaut," *Oklahoma Today* (May 1996), 24 ff.

Wilson, Dorothy Clarke, *Stranger and Traveler: The Story of Dorothea Dix, American Reformer* (New York: Little, Brown and Co., 1975).

Woodham-Smith, Cecil, *Florence Nightingale 1820–1910* (New York: McGraw Hill, 1951).

Woodward, Helen Beal, "The Right to Wear Pants: Dr. Mary Walker," *The Bold Women* (New York: Farrar, Straus and Young, 1953), 281–98.

Zakrzewska, Maria, *A Woman's Quest* (New York: Appleton, 1924).

Zuckerman, Leo, "81-Year-Old Doc Susie Is Fraser's Only Physician," *Rocky Mountain News,* 14 December 1951, 1.

Index

abortion, 19, 26, 32, 37, 74, 75, 183, 184
Adler, Alexandria, 19
Afghanistan, 65
AIDS, 6, 8, 25, 120, 121, 159, 172, 177
Alexander, Virginia, 190
Anderson, Elizabeth Garrett, 100
Anderson, Hedda, 52
Anderson, Susan, 126
Apgar, Virginia, 141
Avishag, Kadari, 50

Badran, Hoda, 66
Baghdad, 67
Barton, Clara, 78
Bassi, Laura, 64
Baumgartner, Leona, 13
Belgium, 55
Berle, Beatrice Bishop, 168, 171
Berman, Elaine, 49
Bickerdyke, Mary Ann, 84
birth control, 26, 37, 40, 63, 75, 120, 183, 184, 185, 187
Blackwell, Elizabeth, 44, 78, 82, 87, 89, 91, 111
Blackwell, Emily, 44
breast cancer, 18, 19, 25, 26
Brown, Dorothy, 189
Bruch, Hilde, 135
Burton, Richard, 69
Bush, George W., 33

Cambel, Perihan, 61
Canadian, 123
Cather, Willa, 27
Chaplin, Matilda, 107
China, 74

Ciller, Tansu, 61
Civil War, 78, 81, 82, 84, 86, 97, 98, 99, 100, 111, 140, 189
Cleveland, Grover, 28
Clinton, Bill, 121, 194
Cole, Rebecca, 96, 190
Collins, Eileen, 195
Cone, Claribel, 137
Conley, Frances, 2
contraceptives. *See* birth control
Cori, Gerty Radnitz, 146
Crumbaker, Deborah, 9
Curie, Marie, 143, 163
Czechoslovakia, 63

Daum, Susan, 13
DeNardo, Sally, 18
Denmark, 54
Denver, 45
Deutsch, Helen, 58
DeVriese, Bertha, 56
Dickey, Nancy Wilson, 1
Dickstein, Leah, 12
Dix, Dorothea, 98
Donne, Maria, 64

Edwards, Brenda, 20
Elders, Joycelyn, 25
Elgood, Sheldon, 69
Elion, Gertrude, 157
Erxleben, Dorothea Leporin, 57
Evans, Helen, 107
Evans, Matilda, 190
Everaert, Clemence, 56

Fenlon, Roberta, 3
fertility rates, 120

Finland, 54
Fisher, Ann, 192
Fleming, Lulu, 190
Folkeson, Maria, 52
Freud, Anna, 58
Freud, Sigmund, 19, 58
Frey, Lucja, 43
Fruchter, Rachel, 8

Garfield, James, 81
Garrett, Mary, 129
Germany, 57
Glassman, Mayera, 51
Gokhan, Nuran, 61
Gorbachev, Mikhail, 63
Greece, 35
Gretsch, Barbara, 10
Grier, Eliza, 190
Gullett, Lucy, 122

Hannikainen, Tingvald, 54
Haseltine, Florence, 21
Hashemi, Fatimeh, 66
Hawks, Esther Hill, 82
Heiken, Rosina, 54
Heim-Vogtlin, Marie, 55
Hemenway, Ruth, 76
Hilliard, Marion, 125
Hittner, Helen, 44
Hodgkin, Dorothy Crowfoot, 148
Holmes, Oliver Wendell, 77
Holth, Marie Spaangberg, 54
Horney, Karen, 58
Horwitz, Susan Band, 4
Hunt, Harriot, 77
Huntington's disease, 177, 179, 180
India, 72
Iran, 66
Israeli women, 47
Italy, 64

Jacobi, Mary Putnam, 110, 129
Jacobs, Aletta, 39
Jacobs, Frances Wisebart, 45
Jalas, Rakel, 54
Japan, 73
Jefferson, Thomas, 168
Jewett, Sarah Orne, 9
Jewish women, 39
Jex-Blake, Sophia, 106
Johnson, Andrew, 83

Johnson, Lyndon, 31, 132
Joshee, Anandabai, 72

Kashevrova-Rudneva, Varvara, 62
Kazim, Mufide, 61
Kelsey, Frances Oldham, 175
Kennedy, John F., 28, 176
Klein, Melanie, 58
Kobayashi, Aya, 73

Lake, Ann Easton, 28
Lawrence, Wendy, 192
Leidenius, Laimi, 54
Lenney, Ruth Kleinfeld, 191
Levi-Montalcini, Rita, 155
Lin, Chiao'chih, 75
Lincoln, Abraham, 83, 84
Lorber, Fannie, 46
Love, Susan, 19
Lucid, Shannon, 193
Lui, Wenxiu, 75

Magora, Florella, 49
Manes, Maria, 167
McClintock, Barbara, 152
Meitner, Lise, 40, 143
Memling Museum, 55
midwife, 35, 37, 39, 57, 62, 67, 68, 69,
    92, 94, 97, 102, 104, 118
Monstavicius, Barbara, 12
Montessori, Maria, 64
Morton, Rosalie Slaughter, 167
Moser, Jana, 63

Netherlands, 55
Niebyl, Jennifer, 134
Nielsen, Nielsine Mathilde, 54
Nightingale, Florence, 89
Norway, 54
Novello, Antonia, 23
Nusslein-Volhard, Christiane, 160
Nyswander, Marie, 172

O'Reilly, Susannah, 121
Okami, Keiko, 73

Pearce, Louise, 132
Pechey, Edith, 107, 110
Pereira-d'Oliverira, E., 55
Pierce-Emerson, Sarah, 190
Pisko, Seraphine Eppstein, 46

Poduslo, Shirley, 20
Polk, Margaret, 76
Preston, Ann, 111

Rabinoff, Sophie, 48
Rahimian, Elham, 66
Ramey, Estelle, 5
Red Cross, 79, 81, 171
Ride, Sally, 63, 192
Robertson, Stella, 138
Roosevelt, Teddy, 78
RU-486, 19
Runge, Nancy, 16
Russia, 62

Sabin, Florence, 130
Safford, Mary, 84
Sanger, Margaret, 184
Santy, Patricia, 192
Saudi Arabia, 67
Saviskaya, Svetlana, 63
Scouros, Maria, 17
Seaman, Jill, 119
Seddon, Rhea, 192
Shakespeare, 23, 143, 189
Shephard, Claudia, 11
SIDS, 15
Smith, Elizabeth, 123
St. Jans Hospital, 55
Stastny, Olga, 64
Stein, Gertrude, 136
Stockton, Sarah, 128
Stopes, Marie, 184, 187
Sudquist, Alma, 52, 53
Sundstrom, Anne, 52
Svartz, Nanna, 53
Sweden, 51
Switzerland, 55
Szold, Henrietta, 47

Tal, Chloe, 48
Taliban, 65
Taussig, Helen, 132, 175
Tereshkova, Valentina, 63
Terzioglu, Meliha, 61
Thorne, Isobel, 110
Thornton, Kathryn, 196
Tiburtius, Franziska, 57
Togasaki, Yoshiye, 138
Toland, Irene, 78
Travell, Janet, 28
Trotula, 39
Tuchman, Barbara, 35
Turkey, 61
Twain, Mark, 77, 183

Valdes-Dapena, Marie, 13
van Diest, Isala, 56
von Bingen, Hildegard, 57

Walker, Mary Edwards, 82, 189
Wallace, Eleanor, 3
Wenger, Nanette, 15
Wexler, Nancy, 177
Whitman, Walt, 89, 129
Widerstrom, Karolina, 52, 53
Williams, Cicely, 116
Willock, Marcelle, 4
Wolf, Jacqueline, 7
Wollstein, Martha, 44
World War I, 146
World War II, 10, 20, 55, 58, 62, 73,
    123, 138, 154, 173, 185, 194

Yalow, Rosalyn, 163
Yoshioka, Yayoi, 73

Zakrzewska, Marie, 97, 111

About the Author

Beatrice Levin set her first published novel, *The Lonely Room,* in Rhode Island and Texas, the two states that have had the greatest influence on her. She is a graduate of Rhode Island College and served in the Women's Army Corps in Texas during World War II. She pursued graduate studies at the University of Wisconsin in English and playwriting. She taught creative writing for more than forty years, and has had fifteen books, more than a thousand articles, and several plays published. Happily married to a scientist for more than fifty years, she is "proud of his significant achievements and those of our three professional sons."